Quick Guide to Dermoscopy in Laser and IPL Treatments

Domenico Piccolo · Dimitra Kostaki
Giuliana Crisman

Quick Guide to Dermoscopy in Laser and IPL Treatments

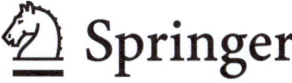 Springer

Domenico Piccolo
Department of Dermatology
University of L'Aquila
AIDA Italian Association Outpatient
Dermatologists AIDA, Avezzano
L'Aquila
Pescara
Italy

Dimitra Kostaki
Sapienza University of Rome
Policlinico Umberto I
Rome
Italy

Giuliana Crisman
Skin Center, Dermo-Aesthetic Centers
Avezzano
Trieste
Italy

ISBN 978-3-319-41632-8   ISBN 978-3-319-41633-5   (eBook)
https://doi.org/10.1007/978-3-319-41633-5

This Springer imprint is published by the registered company Springer Nature Switzerland AG
The registered company address is: Gewerbestrasse 11, 6330 Cham, Switzerland

*I want to dedicate this book
to all the people who have been close
to me over the years
and have helped me in my personal and
professional journey.
A special thanks goes to my mother and
my father
for supporting me in all the difficult
moments of my life.
Thanks to Federica,
an extraordinary wife and mother,
who never leaves me alone and has been my
right arm for 22 years.
To my children, Camilla and Alexandre,
for filling my life with enthusiasm, love,
happiness, and smiles.
To Giuliana and Dimitra,
for their great contribution in writing
this work,
which would not have been possible
without them.*

Domenico Piccolo

*A heartfelt thanks to Domenico
for these years of fruitful collaboration:
if I am now a good laserist, I owe it to him.
To Prof. Ketty Peris,
for all her teachings and for making me a
competent and prepared dermatologist.*

To Giuliana,
for sharing efforts, doubts, articles,
and dreams.
To my parents,
for supporting me at all times,
and to my family,
for always loving me, even if from afar.

Dimitra Kostaki

To my beloved husband Sascha M.,
who has always supported my dreams
and encourages me to follow them.
To my daughter Angelica,
who helps me every day to be a
better woman.
To my mother Margherita,
for her encouragement of all my efforts.
To Domenico,
for giving me the opportunity several times
over the years
to crown a dream, to improve, to learn.
To Dimitra,
for shared evenings full of hope (a few
years ago)
and for the hard work shared (in recent
months).

Giuliana Crisman

Foreword

In an era when new technologies in medicine develop at a rapid pace, few of them finally acquire a real role in clinical practice and even fewer substantially modify it. Dermoscopy is one of them, since its use was adopted by most clinicians all over the world and radically modified the clinical practice of dermatology. Being a small, relatively inexpensive, and fast-to-use tool, the dermatoscope today fits easily in the pocket of most clinicians involved in the diagnosis and management of skin diseases, allowing us to look at submacroscopic features and structures.

After its initial validation for evaluation of skin tumors, the use of dermoscopy with time expanded in more and more fields of dermatology. Light sources (lasers, IPL, etc.) are routinely used by many clinicians around the world for clinical and cosmetic purposes, and the assessment of submacroscopic structures could significantly optimize their use, in terms of evaluating the efficacy as well as the adverse events of the applied treatment. However, as always, the validation of the method represents a cumbersome and long-lasting task.

Having followed the research efforts of the authors of this book during the last years and having the privilege to personally know them, I am really proud of their significant contribution in the field and happy that they decided to undertake the heavy task of putting together all their research and clinical experience in a comprehensive book.

This guide will be useful not only for clinicians who already use dermoscopy to evaluate treatments, but even more for those who never thought about doing it. Filtering their deep knowledge in the topic, the authors provide simple and comprehensive clues and tips that are meant to be applied by all of us, irrespective of our previous experience in dermoscopy.

Therefore, I strongly recommend all colleagues using light devices to not only read this book once but also use it as an everyday guide in their practice.

Aimilio Lallas
First Department of Dermatology
Aristotle University
Thessaloniki, Greece

Preface

I was only a young fellow at the Medical University of Graz when I fell in love with dermoscopy.

I graduated from the University of L'Aquila, not far from where I was born. Professor S. Chimenti, chief of Dermatology Department at the University of L'Aquila, proposed a training period in Graz, Austria, almost 1000 km from home, in order to improve my skills in the field of dermatology and scientific research.

Enthusiastic about the idea of such an important opportunity for professional and personal growth, I left without hesitation.

In Graz, I met who would become my second mentor, Prof. H. P. Soyer, and a young resident, G. Argenziano. That first winter together, under meters of snow, would unite our lives in the research and development of a field that would mark the history of clinical dermatology: Dermoscopy.

Dermoscopy has opened our minds to a new world: studying of skin lesions in their microscopic and structural features, either in normal conditions or in their variations in shape and color. Created to help doctors in differentiating benign lesions from malignant ones, dermoscopy soon proved to be a versatile and promising tool in a wider range of practical applications.

Back home, I became passionate about lasers and pulsed light, their different medical applications, looking for new therapeutic, both effective and fast, painless and without side effects, options for my patients.

Based on my Austrian experience, I applied and amplified all the received teachings, making dermoscopy a pre- and post-treatment diagnostic protocol that I can no longer do without.

In this text, I have collected more than 20 years of experience and clinical cases, and the purpose of this study is to demonstrate the validity of dermoscopy before, during, and after laser and IPL treatment.

All the cases presented in this book have been treated with laser or IPL at our "Skin Center" from 2001 onwards and concern Italian patients with skin types that vary between II and III (according to Fitzpatrick's classification scale). The results obtained therefore concern this type of population. However, I am extremely confident that it will be possible to achieve similar results, with the appropriate adjustments, with skin types of different populations around the world.

L'Aquila, Pescara, Italy   Domenico Piccolo

Contents

Introduction: History, Technique, and Equipment for Dermoscopy

Dermoscopy (also referred elsewhere as dermatoscopy or epiluminescence microscopy) is by definition a noninvasive diagnostic technique for the assessment of skin lesions with an instrument called dermoscope.

The dermoscope is composed of a magnifying glass, a light source (polarized or nonpolarized), a transparent plate, and sometimes a liquid medium (immersion oil, water, alcohol, KY jelly) between the instrument and the skin. The dermoscope allows intra- and sub-epidermic illumination and ensures quick and easy low-cost examinations of skin and mucosal lesions. The term digital epiluminescence dermoscope is also reported in literature when images or videos are acquired or digitally processed.

Dermoscopy has been extensively studied and is widely accepted as a useful tool in dermatological practice. It has been shown that dermoscopy has improved the early diagnosis of malignant melanoma compared to clinical examination only and has subsequently been tested in the diagnosis of different types of skin lesions, which lead to an earlier and more accurate diagnosis avoiding invasive examinations, such as biopsy.

In our daily routine, we tested dermoscopy as a tool for predicting laser and IPL treatment results. Taking advantage of its ability to visualize epidermal structure and superficial dermal structures, a dermoscopic exam, performed immediately before and immediately after a laser session, shows whether the target has been reached and foresees the type of clinical and aesthetic result obtained.

From this point of view, dermoscopy ceases to be merely a diagnostic tool to examine new lesions or to follow up on known lesions and becomes a tool to monitor the effectiveness of the aesthetic and curative treatments performed. The clinician can therefore learn more about the lesion's response to laser treatment, possibly modifying the various parameters and wavelengths to obtain a better result, and therefore the dermoscopic investigation acquires the role of a true ally in dermatological clinical practice.

The contents of this book are partially based on the Italian language edition: *"The Usefulness of Dermoscopy in Laser and IPL Treatments"*, Domenico Piccolo, © DEKA M.E.L.A Srl 2012.

© Springer Nature Switzerland AG 2020
D. Piccolo et al., *Quick Guide to Dermoscopy in Laser and IPL Treatments*,
https://doi.org/10.1007/978-3-319-41633-5_1

1.1   Brief History of Dermoscopy

In the 1930s, several studies on the capillary circulation in healthy and pathological skin (the so-called capillaroscopy) aroused the interest of some authors, who decided to test the use of the in vivo microscope directly on the skin. Particularly, R. and F. Jaeger (1939a, b) and Schmidt-La Baume F. (1940) published three papers to share their results in the study of the skin structure with a direct compound microscope, in which the light entered from the side and was reflected down on the object. Compared to a simple magnifying glass, commonly used in the 1920s and composed of one or more magnifying glasses with a magnification power range from 3× to 200× the capacity of the naked human eye, a compound microscope was better both in resolution, that is in defining the structure of the skin, and in increasing the magnification power up to 40×.

Some years later, Goldman L. and Younker W. (1947a, b) began to study different dermatological conditions with five types of compound microscopes (Fig. 1.1),

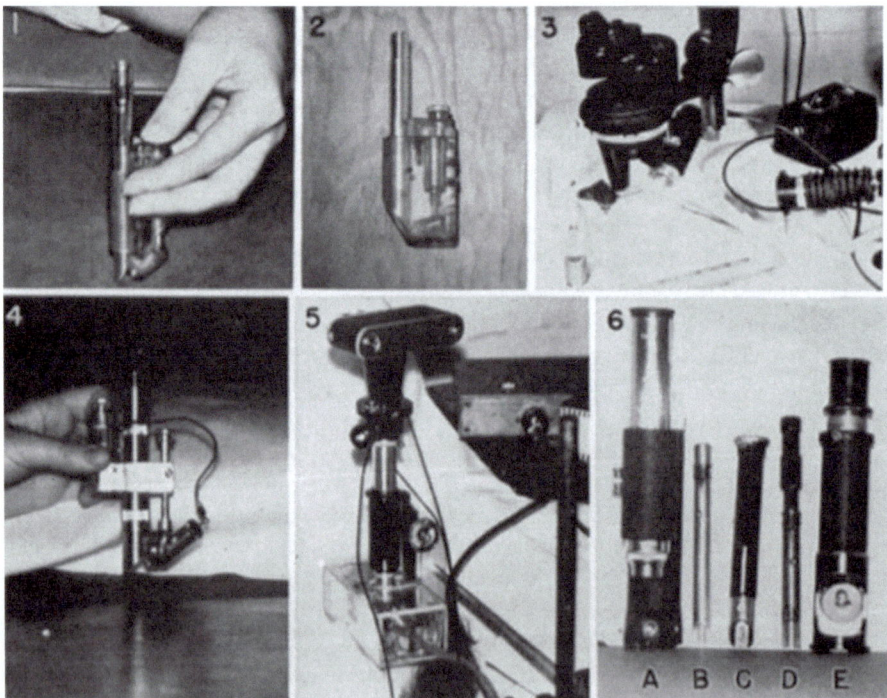

Fig. 1.1 Original instrumentation of cutaneous microscopy (from Goldman. J INVEST DERMATOL 1951, Elsevier license no. 4731201097051)
1. 20× microscope with attached battery illuminator source
2. 40× microscope with simple attached battery illuminator source
3. Technic of examining excised tissue under binocular microscope; illumination can be varied
4. 40× microscope with flexible illumination source
5. Photomicrographic apparatus of Siebentritt for photography of surface of skin at magnifications of 40× and 100×

with and without light and/or with and without fluorescent lighting, and tried to improve these equipment in order to apply dermoscopy to the study of normal and pathological skin.

Subsequently, Goldman (1951) focused on the study of pigmented lesions in order to help the doctor in the difficult differential diagnosis between dysplastic nevi and early melanoma and published his results on 300 melanocytic lesions. He also emphasized the need for a portable instrument, since all the tested microscopes are promising in the result, but difficult to manage, so in 1952 he invented the first portable dermoscope, a prototype subsequently developed and improved. But it was only in 1987, with the studies of Pehamberger and his collaborators (1987), that dermoscopy acquired its specific and fundamental role in the diagnosis of pigmented lesions as we know it today (Fig. 1.2).

In 1989, Hamburg hosted the first consensus meeting on dermoscopy, in which the first common terminology for dermoscopic criteria was established. Some years later, Nachbar F and his colleagues (1996) proposed the first semiquantitative diagnostic algorithm, the so-called ABCD rule of dermatoscopy, while in 1998 Argenziano and his collaborators (1998) introduced the "7-point checklist" as a semiquantitative diagnostic system, based on a simplified analysis of the lesion model.

Fig. 1.2 The microscope used in the study of Pehamberger et al. in 1987 for the examination of pigmented skin lesions in a patient both in upright and supine positions. (J Am Acad Dermatol 1987, Elsevier license no. 4731210028901)

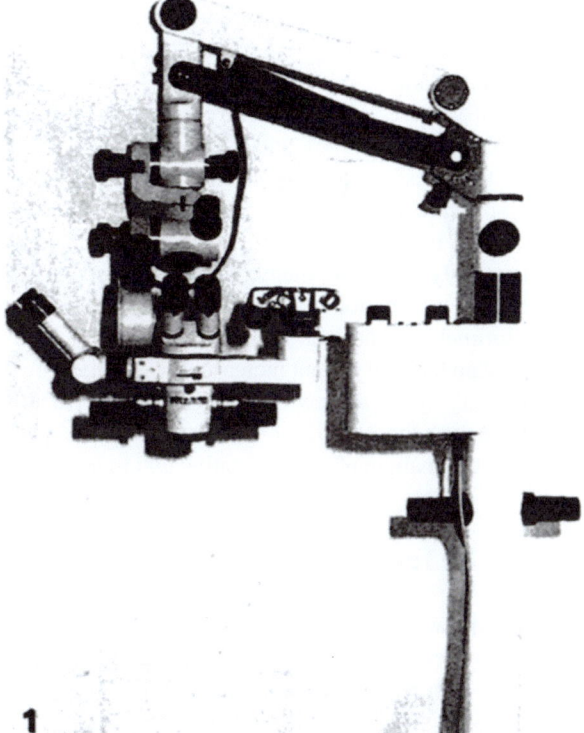

With the advent of the new millennium, another milestone was set in the history of dermoscopy, with the publication of the first interactive atlas of CD-ROM dermoscopy, in which the main diagnostic criteria were defined by Argenziano and collaborators.

From that moment on, dermoscopy has become a significant part of dermatological practice, so that in 2003 Peter Soyer, Rainer Hofmann-Wellenhof, and Giuseppe Argenziano founded the International Dermoscopy Society, in order to promote dermoscopy in clinical research, development, and dissemination in the world. So far (2019), IDS has over 16,000 members in 168 different countries (https://dermoscopy-ids.org).

Created with the aim of improving diagnostics in dermatology, with the development of new devices for medical and aesthetic therapy, dermoscopy is taking on an important new role in monitoring results and in the faster identification of possible relapses, as will be explained more in detail in this volume.

1.2   The Equipment

Nowadays, the required equipment consists at least of a dermoscope and a camera connected to a software, in order to acquire and archive all the acquired images.

The dermoscope is a mono-ocular instrument composed of a head and a handpiece. The head is composed of a halogen or led lamp for lighting and a magnifying glass: a spherical lens with a fixed 10× magnification. The instrument is connected to a digital camera, which can then be connected to a PC for a software analysis of the collected data.

Currently, there are many different types of dermoscopes (with or without polarizing light, for example) and numerous accessories (special adapters to reach difficult-to-access anatomical sites, adapters for mobile cameras, etc.) (Fig. 1.3).

The software improves the quality of the evaluation of suspected skin lesions (in particular, in the differential diagnosis of dysplastic nevus and early melanoma) by simultaneously analyzing many clinical microscopic data, therefore not detectable by a naked eye examination but also by the mere use of the dermoscope, as morphometric and colorimetric examinations. The capability to view, document, and archive all images taken by each patient increases the quality of follow-up. Thanks to the possibility of identifying the microscopic lesion changes (in terms of dimensions, edges, color, and so on) over time, the dermatologist may be able to promptly intervene both in the case of initial malignant transformation and in the case of post-treatment relapses.

1.3   The Technique

Dermoscopy was originated as a second-level clinical investigation, since it is subsequent to a clinical evaluation of the patient. Once a suspicious lesion has been identified, a macroscopic evaluation is performed, evaluating the various characteristics (such as size, color, edges, symmetry, etc.) visible to the naked eye.

Fig. 1.3 (**a**, **b**) Portable
dermoscope connected to a
smartphone. (Courtesy of
Dr. Domenico Piccolo,
Skin Center
Avezzano, Italy)

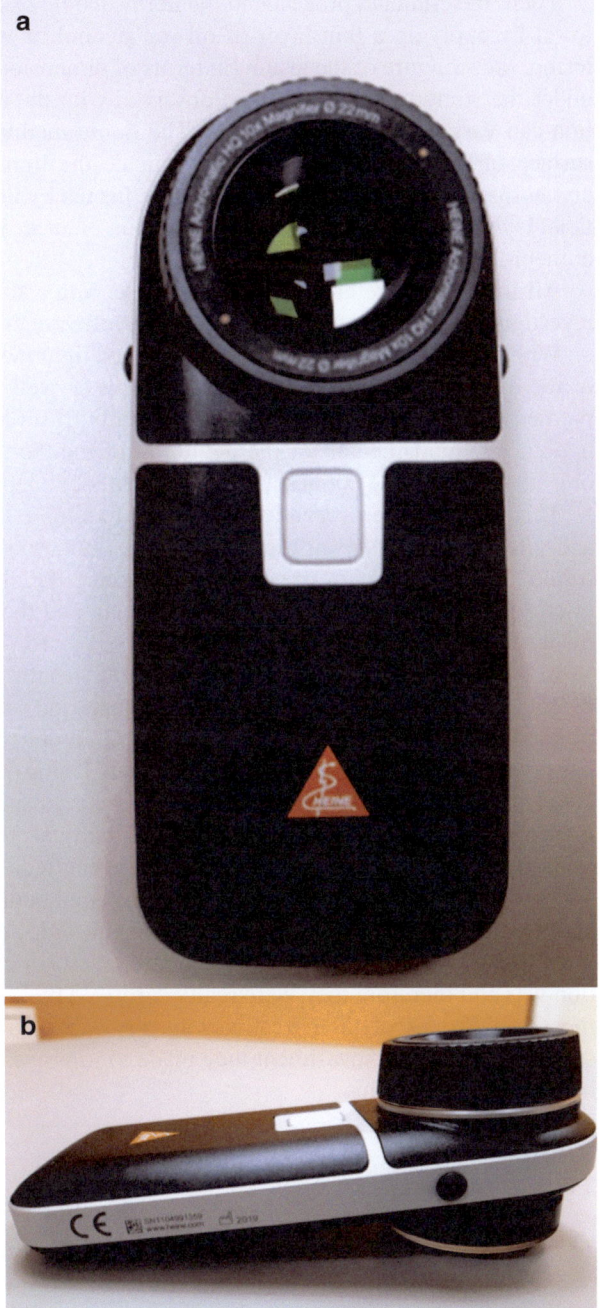

Then, the clinician proceeds to the dermoscopic examination, performed as follows: by applying a thin layer of oil (or alcohol or water) on the identified skin lesion, the structure of the lesion (in terms of dimensions, edges, color, etc.) located under the stratum corneum can be observed with the dermoscope. The magnification can vary between 6× and 400×. The liquid medium between the lens and the surface of the skin is necessary to eliminate the light reflected from the stratum corneum: the light beam is absorbed and reflected by the structure under that superficial layer, thus leading to a better inspection of each structure between the stratum corneum and the dermo-epidermal junction.

All images that refer to skin lesions deserving a strict follow-up and/or further investigation are collected, analyzed by the software, and archived.

With the advent of the new laser and pulsed light methodologies in the treatment of the most common dermatological diseases as well as in the treatment of some pigmented lesions, a tool was needed not only to formulate the correct diagnostic hypothesis, fundamental for the definition of the therapeutic protocol, but also to objectively assess the initial state and the result obtained at the end of each treatment.

This role had been previously entrusted to simple clinical photographs "before and after treatment", even though with the limitations of highlighting only great results, since the images are not able to notice the slightest changes, sometimes microscopic, appreciated by both the clinician and the patient, between one treatment session and another.

In this volume, we have tried to share our results in testing dermoscopy as a diagnostic and follow-up tool for all our patients and we have established a rigorous protocol to scientifically validate this method. In our routine practice, dermoscopy has proved to be very accurate not only for the diagnosis of the lesions to be treated, but also to predict and quantify any damage and adverse events. Furthermore, dermoscopic examination was mandatory in a clinical follow-up session 4–6 weeks after treatment for all nonmelanoma skin cancers treated with laser and IPL-PDT.

Moreover, thanks to this precise iconographic documentation, the patients were able to observe and appreciate the results achieved, also because in an interval of 4–6 months of treatment they often did not remember exactly what the initial situation was and therefore they were really surprised by seeing all the clinical and dermoscopic images of their treatment history. This obviously contributed to their satisfaction with the investment they made to improve their conditions, in terms of both economy and time.

1.4   Teledermoscopy

At the end of the 1900s, advances in computer technology gave rise to the introduction of a revolutionary diagnostic method known as "telemedicine." Its use in various medical disciplines involves the communication and exchange not only of scientific information but also the possibility of sending requests for second opinions to other sites (virtually anywhere in the world) with short waiting times, allowing an almost immediate diagnosis and reducing costs for the health system.

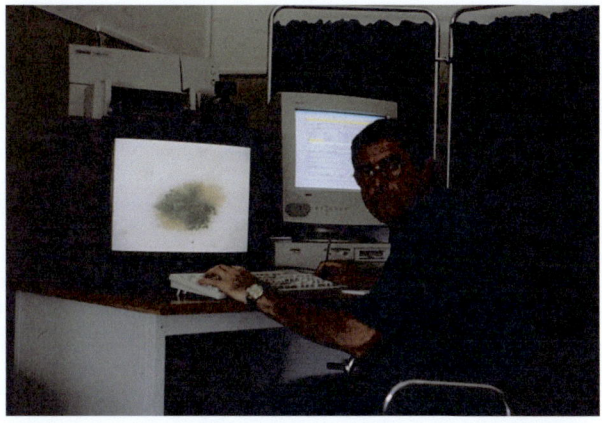

Fig. 1.4 Prof. S. Chimenti during the first pioneering study on teledermoscopy (1996–1999): selection of the dermoscopic images at the University of L'Aquila (L'Aquila, Italy), subsequently sent by email to the Medical University of Graz (Graz, Austria). (Courtesy of Dr. Domenico Piccolo, Skin Center Avezzano, Italy)

In all departments where a precise assessment in such difficult cases is important for diagnosis and treatment, telemedicine could become an integral part of daily practice.

Dermatology and in particular dermatoscopy could greatly benefit from telemedicine because the application of teledermoscopy allows you to contact specialists and experts from all over the world, perform comparative analyzes and statistical studies, thus obtaining economic and social benefits.

Domenico Piccolo, along with his mentors, including S. Chimenti, H.P. Soyer, and R. Hofmann-Wellenhof, was one of the pioneers in the possible applications of telemedicine in dermatoscopy. In 1999, Piccolo D. et al. (1999) published the first study in teledermoscopy: 66 pigmented skin lesions were examined clinically from an en face view at the Dermatology Clinical Department of L'Aquila (L'Aquila, Italy). Clinical and dermoscopic image of each lesion have been picked and all data (together with clinical data) have been sent via email on a standard resolution color monitor (Fig. 1.4) for consultation at the Dermatology Department of the Medical University of Graz (Graz, Austria). The authors demonstrated a diagnostic concordance in 91% of cases (60/66 lesions): a first important milestone was set in the evolution of teledermoscopy, which has since become a fundamental tool of medical practice and used throughout the world.

Nowadays, telemedicine is a consolidated and widespread reality, which allows doctors all over the world to improve the quality of health care provided.

References

Argenziano G, Fabbroccini G, Carlo P, et al. Epiluminescence microscopy for the diagnosis of doubtful melanocytic lesions. Comparison of the ABCD rule of dermatoscopy and a new 7-point checklist based on pattern analysis. Arch Dermatol. 1998;134:1563–70.

Goldman L. Some investigative studies of pigmented nevi with cutaneous microscopy. J Invest Dermatol. 1951;16:407–26.

Goldman L, Younker W. Studies in microscopy of the surface of the skin. J Invest Dermatol. 1947a;9:11.

Goldman L, Younker W. Clinical microscopy of the surface of the skin. Exhibit A.M.A., Atlantic City; 1947b.

Jaeger R, Jaeger F. Fluoreszenzmikroskopie in Auffallenden Licht unter besonderer Berücksichtigung der Struktur der Oberflache der lebenden Haut und der Vereinfachung der Hilfsmittel. Ztschr, f wissensch Mikr. 1939a;56:273.

Jaeger R, Jaeger F. Der Haut Oberflaschenstruktur. Arch f Gewerbepath u Gewerbehyg. 1939b;9:276.

Nachbar F, Stolz W, Merkel T, et al. ABCD rule of dermatoscopy. J Am Acad Dermatol. 1996;13:91–2.

Pehamberger H, Steiner A, Wolff K. In vivo epiluminescence microscopy of pigmented skin lesions. I. Pattern analysis of pigmented skin lesions. J Am Acad Dermatol. 1987;17(4):571–83.

Piccolo D, Smolle J, Wolf IH, et al. Face-to-face diagnosis vs telediagnosis of pigmented skin tumors: a teledermoscopic study. Arch Dermatol. 1999;135(12):1467–71.

Schmidt-LaBaume F. Die Bedeutung der Fuloreszenzauflicht und Kapillar Mikroskopie fur Gewerbliche Hauterkrankugen. Zermatt Wchnshr. 1940;110:81.

Lasers in Dermatology: Basic Principles 2

LASER stands for Light Amplification by Stimulated Emission of Radiation and refers to instruments designed to emit specific light beams. A LASER device is designed to emit monochromatic light, coherent light, or collimated light in order to obtain different results when interacting with tissues.

For example, a monochromatic light is made up of a single wavelength that is strictly specific to a tissue target or a chromophore (such as melanin or hemoglobin), thus avoiding any damage to surrounding structures.

A device with a coherent light is a laser in which light waves move in the spatial and temporal phases, creating coherence that optimizes the interaction of the beam with human tissues, whereas a laser with a collimated light source is a device with a lens system with different focal lengths mounted on articulated arms that concentrate the laser beam emitted on very small spots (Patil and Dhami 2008; Sebaratnam et al. 2014).

To better understand the light–tissue interactions some terms must be defined:

- Wavelength
- Thermal Relaxation Time (TRT)
- Pulse Duration and Pulse Delay
- Laser Output Power and Beam Diameter (Energy Density)

2.1 Wavelength

The most important parameter to set is represented by the wavelength, because some wavelengths are selectively absorbed by specific molecules present in the skin and defined as "targets" or chromophores (such as water, melanin, hemoglobin) (Fig. 2.1). This absorption generates a large amount of heat in the target (by

---

The contents of this book are partially based on the Italian language edition: "*The Usefulness of Dermoscopy in Laser and IPL Treatments*", Domenico Piccolo, © DEKA M.E.L.A Srl 2012.

© Springer Nature Switzerland AG 2020
D. Piccolo et al., *Quick Guide to Dermoscopy in Laser and IPL Treatments*,
https://doi.org/10.1007/978-3-319-41633-5_2

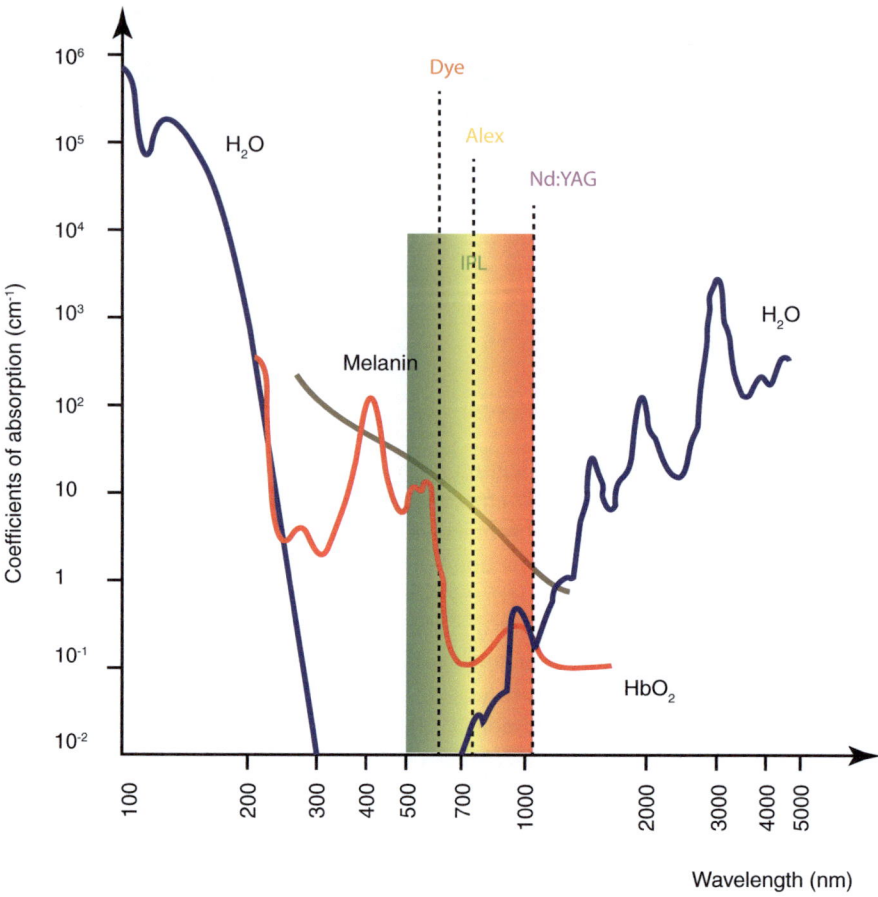

Fig. 2.1 Cutaneous chromophores and their wavelengths. (Courtesy of DEKA M.E.L.A. S.r.l.)

conversion of the radiant energy light into thermal energy), which is able to selectively destroy the target molecules (selective photothermolysis), with minimal damage to the surrounding tissues (Anderson and Parrish 1983; Margolis et al. 1989).

The penetration depth of the visible light increases with increasing wavelength. Penetration of short wavelength (300–400 nm) into the skin is limited, while longer wavelengths (1000–1200 nm) allow the light to reach a depth of even 4 mm due to their increased diffusion. In the visible range, the most important chromophores are melanin and hemoglobin (Anderson and Parrish 1983). Laser for vascular and photorejuvenation treatments should be used in this range.

Moreover, in the infrared range, water, which is the main component of the skin, plays a fundamental role in the laser–tissue interaction (Fig. 2.2). Er:YAG and CO_2 lasers emit in the infrared spectrum (at a 2940 and 10,600 nm wavelength) where absorption of the radiation by the water molecules prevails over penetration (Boyce and Alster 2002).

Fig. 2.2 Laser-tissue
interaction. (Courtesy of
DEKA M.E.L.A. S.r.l.)

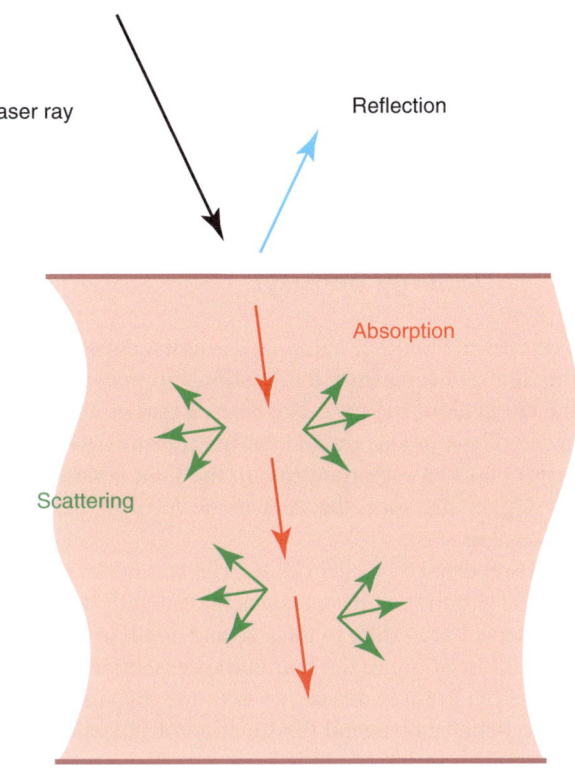

2.2   Thermal Relaxation Time (TRT)

By definition, thermal relaxation time is the time taken by an object (in this case, a
biological structure) to cool down to 50% of its original temperature. Cooling can
be achieved by convection, radiation, and conduction, even though the latter remains
still the main component.

2.3   Pulse Duration and Pulse Delay

The destructive capacity of a laser also depends largely on the duration of the light
pulse it is capable of emitting. After heating, any biological structure releases heat
to cool down and it takes some time; therefore, selective destruction (Selective
Photothermolysis theory) can be obtained only if the duration of the laser pulse is
less than the TRT (Anderson and Parrish 1983).

Pulse delivery with a shorter duration than TRT allows limiting thermal damage
to the target set and minimizes the spread of heat to adjacent tissues. The TRT of
large targets is longer than the TRT of the smaller chromophores. Consequently, the
possibility of programming the duration of the laser energy pulse based on the size

of the chromophores is essential for an accurate treatment of the lesion, preventing damage to the surrounding tissues, and minimizing the risks of scarring.

If *Pulse Duration* represents the time of exposure to the light beam, *Pulse Delay* represents the time that the skin and blood vessels need to cool down between pulses, while the heat is retained inside the target.

2.4   Laser Output Power and Beam Diameter (Energy Density)

The effects of a laser beam on the tissue depend on the concentration of photons in the light ray (i.e., from the relationship between the poor output of the device and the diameter of the ray). The beam's size of an instrument is important both for the speed of the procedure and for the transmission. The size of the device spot (footprint) plays an important role in the light penetration into the tissue. Synthetically, the bigger the spot, the deeper the level of penetration (Carroll and Humphreys 2006) (Fig. 2.3).

As reported by Keijzer et al. (1989), a better efficacy and a more planar geometry of light penetration have been achieved with larger footprint. The spot's size should be selected according to the size and depth of the lesion. For example, the transmission of laser light to the hair bulb is essential for deep follicular damage and as the size of the beam increases, so does the transmission.

To better understand the function of the various types of laser it is necessary to know the meaning of terms such as power, energy, and density.

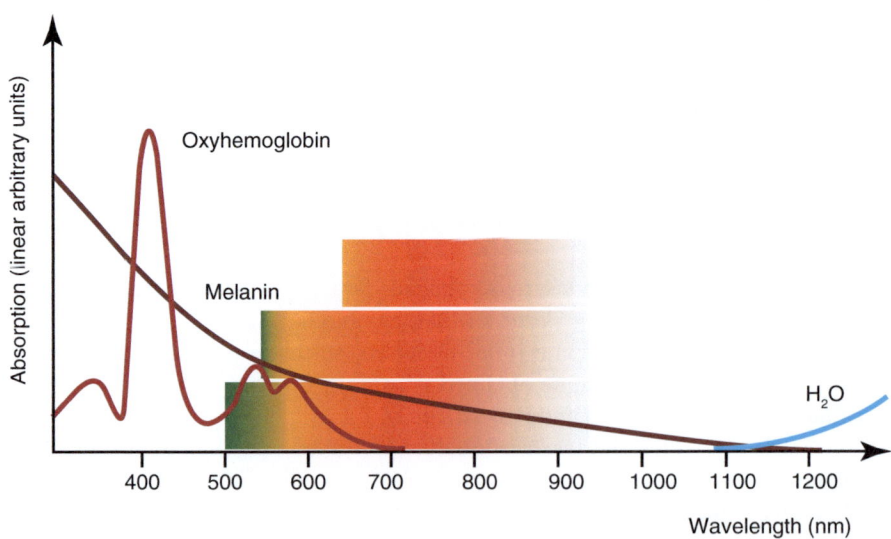

Fig. 2.3 Use of filters to block the undesired wavelengths. (Courtesy of DEKA M.E.L.A. S.r.l.)

- *Energy* is expressed in Joules and represents the number of photons produced during the emission of the pulse.
- *Power* is expressed in Watts and represents the number of photons emitted in a specific unit of time.
- *Fluence* or energy density is expressed in Joule/square centimeter and represents the number of photons produced during the emission of the pulse in the area radiated by the laser beam.

To obtain the correct thermal effects of light on human skin, it is also necessary to consider the damage caused to the tissues by the temperature reached.

References

Anderson RR, Parrish JA. Selective photothermolysis: precise microsurgery by selective absorption of pulsed irradiation. Science. 1983;22:524–7.

Boyce S, Alster TS. CO2 laser treatment of epidermal nevi: long-term success. Dermatol Sure. 2002;28:611–4.

Carroll L, Humphreys TR. LASER-tissue interactions. Clin Dermatol. 2006;24(1):2–7.

Keijzer M, Jacques SL, Prahl SA, et al. Light distributions in artery tissue: Monte Carlo simulations for finite-diameter laser beams. Lasers Sure Med. 1989;9(2):148–54.

Margolis RJ, Dover JS, Polla LL, et al. Visible action spectrum for melanin-specific selective photothermolysis. Lasers Surg Med. 1989;9.389–97.

Patil UA, Dhami LD. Overview of lasers. Indian J Plast Surg. 2008;41(Suppl):S101–13.

Sebaratnam DF, Lim AC, Lowe PM, et al. Lasers and laser-like devices: part two. Aust J Dermatol. 2014;55:1–14.

Laser–Tissue Interactions

3

Laser and IPL therapies have found remarkable success in the dermatological field due to the satisfactory results achieved (Raulin et al. 2003; Tanzi et al. 2003; Patil and Dhami 2008).

In this chapter, we will describe the interactions between lasers and IPLs with tissues, such as skin and mucous membranes.

To better understand how light beams interact with skin and mucous membrane (such as lips, for instance), it is mandatory to describe how these tissues are composed.

3.1 Histopathology of the Skin

Skin histopathology, also called dermatopathology, is surprisingly complex because many different types of cells are involved, interacting with each other in order to ensure several important functions, from photo protection to mechanical barrier, from immunosurveillance to nutrient metabolism.

The skin originates from the ectoderm, which is one of the three embryonic leaflets and represents the outermost primitive germinal layer of the embryo (distal layer). The other two layers are the mesoderm (middle layer) and the endoderm (proximal layer). In vertebrates, the ectoderm has three parts: external ectoderm (also known as superficial ectoderm), the neural crest, and the neural tube. The last two layers are also known as neuroectoderm.

The ectoderm gives rise to the skin epidermis and its derived structures, internal epithelial lining of the mouth and rectum, sensory epidermal receptors, cornea and crystalline, adrenal medullary, tooth enamel, dermal bones, and finally the nervous tissue, through a process known as neurulation.

In humans, it appears during the third week during embryogenesis. After the formation of the endoderm and the intra-embryonic mesoderm, the epiblast takes

The contents of this book are partially based on the Italian language edition: "*The Usefulness of Dermoscopy in Laser and IPL Treatments*", Domenico Piccolo, © DEKA M.E.L.A Srl 2012.

© Springer Nature Switzerland AG 2020   15
D. Piccolo et al., *Quick Guide to Dermoscopy in Laser and IPL Treatments*,
https://doi.org/10.1007/978-3-319-41633-5_3

the name of ectoderm, thus constituting the last of the three sheets of the embryonic trilaminar disk.

The skin is generally divided into two separate but functionally interdependent layers: epidermis and dermis (Fig. 3.1). Although it is not part of the skin, subcutaneous adipose tissue is usually evaluated by the dermatologist, because it usually tends to respond together with the skin in many pathological processes.

The epidermis is mainly composed of the following:

- *Keratinocytes* (over 90%): their primary function is the formation of a barrier against environmental damage (i.e., bacteria, viruses, fungi, parasites, but also physical damage such as heat, UV radiation, and, at least, water loss).
- *Melanocytes*: they product melanin, a dark pigment primarily responsible for skin color (and subsequently for pigmentary disorders) (Fig. 3.2). Once synthesized, melanin is contained in melanosomes, special organelles that can be transported to nearby keratinocytes to induce pigmentation. Functionally, melanin serves as a protection against UV radiation. Melanocytes play also a role in the immune system.
- *Langerhans cells* are present in all layers of the epidermis and are most prominent in the stratum spinosum. They also occur in the papillary dermis, particularly around blood vessels, as well as in the oral mucosa, foreskin, and vaginal epithelium. They exploit an immunity function by processing microbial antigens, thus becoming fully functional APC (antigen presenting cells).

Fig. 3.1 Histological section of normal skin in hematoxylin & eosin stain for microscopic examination (20×). (Courtesy of Dr. Simonetta Battocchio, Pathology Unit, Spedali Civili of Brescia, Brescia, Italy)

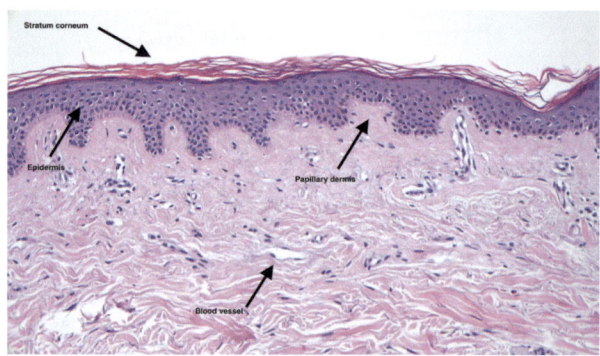

Fig. 3.2 Basal cells with melanin (arrows, Orcein stain, 40×). (Courtesy of Dr. Simonetta Battocchio, Pathology Unit, Spedali Civili of Brescia, Brescia, Italy)

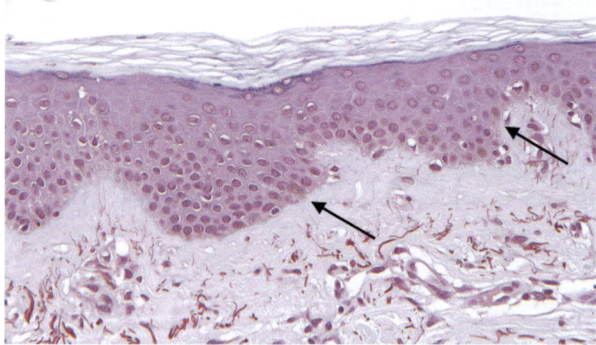

Fig. 3.3 Orcein stain
highlights the dermal
content of elastin within
the dermis (20×).
(Courtesy of Dr. Simonetta
Battocchio, Pathology
Unit, Spedali Civili of
Brescia, Brescia, Italy)

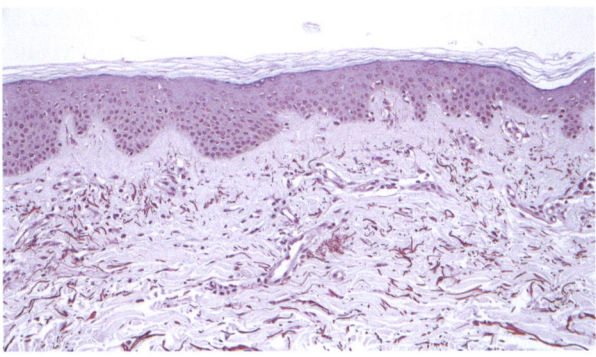

- *Merkel cells*, also known as Merkel–Ranvier cells or tactile epithelial cells, are oval-shaped mechanoreceptors essential for light touch sensation and found in the skin of vertebrates.
- *Toker cells* (putatively programmed for a possible annexed/glandular differentiation in the nipple area in about 10% of individuals).
- *Unmyelinated axons*.

The epidermis shows a particular architecture, with an undulant undersurface visible in two-dimensional sections, with downward invaginations termed rotes and interdigitating mesenchymal cones called dermal papillae.

Separated from the epidermis by the dermoepidermal junctions, composed of particular types of cellular junctions which are involved in several dermatological conditions (i.e., pemphigo and pemphigoides), the dermis is a complex tissue composed of fibroblasts, dendritic and nondendritic monocytes/macrophages, factor XIIIa-expressing dermal dendrocytes, and mast cells, which are developed within a matrix of collagen and glycosaminoglycan, in which it is possible to recognize adnexal and vascular structures and elastic fibers (Fig. 3.3).

3.2   Laser–Tissue Interactions: From Lasers to IPL

The main goal when using a pulsed surgical laser is to obtain ablation by minimizing heat damage. This can be achieved by vaporizing the tissue for less time than is necessary for heat propagation (a time less than TRT).

To obtain instant ablation, the energy of the laser beam must exceed the vaporization threshold of the skin, below which the only effect will be the carbonization and necrosis of the tissue. This consideration is fundamental for the correct use of surgical lasers: the minimum heat damage is obtained with high-power and ultra-short pulses. Depending on the degree and time of exposure of the tissues, this effect can be divided into three different mechanisms:

- *Hyperthermia*, which leads to a moderate increase in temperature (only a few degrees Celsius) above normal physiological conditions for several minutes (temperatures between 41 and 44 °C).

- *Coagulation*, which is obtained with exposure to temperatures between 50 and 90 °C for one second at a time, producing desiccation and shrinkage of the tissue due to the denaturation of tissue proteins, including collagen. The treated tissues are removed by the operator (debridement) and the repair process begins. Coagulation is used to destroy tissues and stop bleeding (hemostasis).
- *Vaporization*, which leads to an immediate loss of substances in the tissues. The different constituents of the tissues are eliminated at temperatures above 300 °C for a relatively short time (a few tenths of a second). If an extremely high temperature can be reached in a very short time, it will be possible to obtain the vaporization of the target with scarce or absent necrosis at the margins of the lesion. This phenomenon, called photoablation, involves a minimally explosive photodecomposition.

As we described in the previous chapter, some wavelengths are selectively absorbed by targets or chromophores such as melanin and hemoglobin. Melanin is produced by melanocytes present in the epidermis, while hemoglobin is contained in the erythrocytes that circulate in the capillaries of the superficial vascular plexuses of the dermis (Polla et al. 1987).

This is why the technological interest has focused on the development of medical devices capable of intervening on particular skin conditions, precisely exploiting these two target molecules present in the epidermis and dermis, respectively (Tanzi et al. 2003) (Fig. 3.4).

Laser and IPL therapies have proven to be the most important and accurate treatments for the removal of pigmented chromatic alterations of various benign effects.

Fig. 3.4 Penetration of the skin by light beam depending on its wavelength. (Courtesy of DEKA M.E.L.A. S.r.l.)

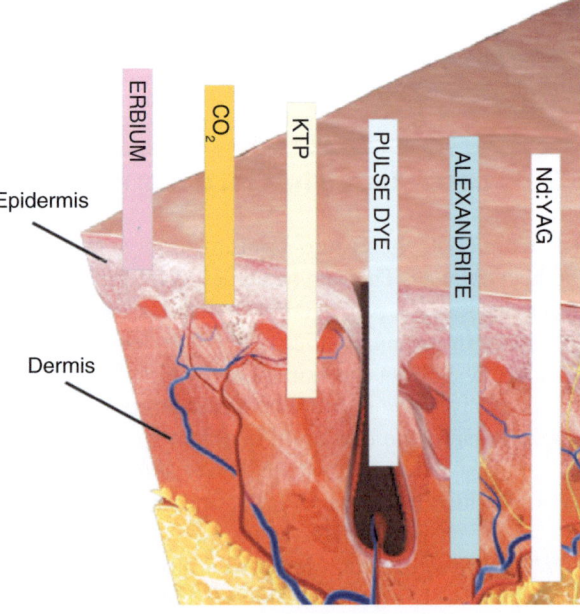

This goal has been reached only with the latest generation of light-based technologies, capable of limiting thermal damage to the chromophores responsible for pigmentation by acting selectively on the wavelength, and with optimal management of the pulse duration (Fitzpatrick et al. 1993; Bukvić Mokos et al. 2010).

First described by Anderson and Parrish, the theory of selective photothermolysis revolutionized laser therapy by establishing a protocol of producing localized tissue damage sparing the surrounding tissue (Anderson and Parrish 1983).

Melanin, a substance contained in melanosomes within the epidermis and dermoepidermal junction (horizontal distribution of melanin), is the chromophore target of pigmented lesions. Furthermore, it is highly concentrated in hair follicles and in the vertical growth components of melanocytic nevi (Polla et al. 1987).

Melanin has a broad and intense absorption spectrum through ultraviolet, visible, and near-infrared spectra (Anderson and Parrish 1983). To obtain selective photothermolysis of melanin, it is necessary to use light sources with wavelengths that are both preferably absorbed by melanin compared to other skin chromophores, such as hemoglobin, and penetrate to the desired depth. Therefore, lasers that emit wavelengths of 630–1100 nm can provide selective absorption of melanosomes, good skin penetration, and selection of melanin on hemoglobin.

Through this wide range of wavelengths, hypothetically any laser with sufficient energy levels can affect melanin. However, the differences in the nature of the target pigment (endogenous or exogenous pigment), in its absorption characteristics, in its distribution within the tissue (intracellular or extracellular), and in its anatomical position in the skin (epidermal, dermal or both) have led to a wide spectrum of results obtained between different types of lasers (Stratigos et al. 2000).

A logical and systematic approach for laser removal of benign pigmented lesions is to classify them according to the position of the abnormal pigment.

Benign pigmented lesions are usually classified into three groups, namely (1) epidermal pigmented lesions (including solar lentigo, ephelides, café au lait macules, and seborrheic keratoses); (2) dermal lesions (such as melanocytic nevi, blue nevi, drug-induced hyperpigmentation, and nevus of Ota and Ito); and (3) mixed (epidermal/dermal) pigmented lesions (such as Becker's nevus, postinflammatory hyperpigmentation, melasma, and nevus spilus).

In current practice, there are several lasers that can specifically target pigmented lesions, and they are classified into three categories: (1) green-light lasers (e.g., 510-nm pulsed dye, 532-nm frequency-doubled Nd:YAG), (2) red-light lasers (e.g., 694-nm ruby, 755-nm alexandrite), and (3) near-infrared lasers (e.g., 1064 nm Nd:YAG). Green-light lasers can be pulse or continuous wave. Red-light lasers are divided into short and long pulse systems. The near-infrared laser currently available is short pulsed. The shorter wavelengths (<600 nm) require relatively less energy fluences, while at longer wavelengths higher fluences are required to produce an effective photothermal reaction (Margolis et al. 1989). Green-light lasers are therefore more effective in treating epidermal pigmented lesions, thanks to their ability to optically penetrate very little into the skin layers and to require relatively less energy to produce irreversible thermal damage to melanosomes (Fitzpatrick et al. 1993; Patel 1998; Hamilton 2004).

In contrast, red-light and near-infrared lasers are more successful in treating deeper dermal melanosomes, i.e., dermal lesions due to their longer wavelengths (Bukvić Mokos et al. 2010).

To achieve a selective destruction of melanin, pulse duration represents a fundamental tool. The selection of the pulse duration is mainly guided by the size of the target and its TRT (thermal relaxation time). In general, the optimal pulse width should be shorter than the TRT of the intended target structure. This ensures that the energy is delivered to the melanin only in the target lesion and does not have sufficient time to extend to the surrounding tissue (Castanet and Ortonne 1997).

With an estimated relaxation time ranging from 250 to 1000 ns, depending on their size, melanosomes require submicrosecond laser pulses for their selective interruption. Therefore, short pulse lasers with pulse durations of 40–750 ns are used, while longer pulse durations, in milliseconds, do not cause specific damage to melanosomes, since melanosomes cool off before adjacent structures without providing the expected results and instead causing serious thermal damage to the surrounding tissue (Vejjabhinanta et al. 2010). In many pigmented lesions, however, melanosomes and melanocytes are clustered so compactly that they act as a larger body than chromophore. In this situation, even the specific wavelengths of melanin in milliseconds lead to the clearance of the lesion (Patil and Dhami 2008).

According to the literature, subnanosecond domain (femtosecond and picosecond) pulse width lasers have been introduced in an attempt to achieve even more effective pigment destruction with even less damage to the surrounding tissue, but their results are still controversial (Stratigos et al. 2000; Kasai 2017).

Taking into account the above, the most specific lasers currently available for the treatment of benign pigmented lesions are short pulse lasers, Q-switched (QS) lasers (nanosecond and picosecond lasers) that exhibit both photothermal and photomechanical effects (Watanabe et al. 1987). Four types of short pulse QS lasers are currently available in clinical use today: the QS ruby laser (694 nm, 25–40 ns), the QS (755 nm, 50–100 ns), the QS Nd:YAG (1064 nm, 5–10 ns), and frequency-doubled Nd:YAG (532 nm, 5–10 ns).

Superficial lesions are more suitable for shorter wavelengths (532 QS Nd:YAG, QS ruby) (Taylor et al. 1993). For lesions where pigment is deposited more deeply in the dermis and for darker skin types (III–IV), it is necessary to select a longer wavelength, making the QS Nd:YAG at 1064 nm the ideal laser to use (Taylor and Anderson 1993).

The mechanism proposed behind the destruction of melanosomes by these lasers is that the thermal confinement of visible radiation at high intensity and short pulse generates acoustic waves by thermal expansion, leading to mechanical damage to the cells (Ara et al. 1990). Tissue repair following laser-induced melanosomal disruption demonstrates an initial two-stage transient skin depigmentation followed by subsequent repigmentation weeks later (Fitzpatrick et al. 1993).

Other pigment-specific lasers like argon (488 and 514 nm), krypton (520–530 nm), and copper vapor (511 nm) can also be effective in the hands of experienced operators (Apfelberg et al. 1979; Dinehart et al. 1993; Skobelkin et al. 1989; Patel 1998).

However, their use has been limited in recent years due to the increased incidence of side effects compared to QS lasers. In particular, these lasers operate in continuous or quasi-continuous wave mode. Thus, although they selectively target melanin, the thermal lesion does not remain limited to the target but dissipates in the surrounding tissues, increasing the risk of hypopigmentation and scarring (Apfelberg et al. 1981). Furthermore, due to their shorter wavelengths, these lasers do not penetrate very deeply into the dermis and are therefore ineffective for the treatment of pigmented dermal lesions.

Ablative lasers like carbon dioxide (CO_2, 10,600 nm) and Er:YAG (2940 nm) with water as a target chromophore in epidermis have been also tested to treat superficial pigmented lesions, especially thicker and hyperkeratotic ones, as seborrheic keratosis, and "Q-switched resistant" Café-Au-Lait macules (Patil and Dhami 2008; Hamilton 2004; Boyce and Alster 2002). These devices exert their effect by stripping the epidermis with consequent damage to the pigments. Furthermore, it has been reported that ablative lasers are quite effective in removing skin-colored skin nevi (Hammes et al. 2008; Sardana 2013). In particular, shave excision along with CO_2 re-contouring of these nevi is an accepted clinical practice due to low risk of malignant transformation (Sebaratnam et al. 2014). Although excellent cosmetic outcomes can be achieved with ablative lasers, nonselective destruction can lead to post-treatment erythema, infection, and possible pigmentary and structural/textural changes. The risk of these complications is, however, minimized with the most recent short pulse systems due to the controlled heating of tissues (Boyce and Alster 2002). In fact, instead of producing a continuous wave, the ultra-pulsed devices produce high energy and ultra-short pulses of laser light, ensuring that the TRT of the target tissues is not exceeded. This allows the user to accurately remove lesions with minimal charring and thermal injury to surrounding tissues.

The CO_2 laser (carbon dioxide laser) is widely used in dermatological practice and TRT (as previously reported, the time taken by a biological structure to lose 50% of its heat) is essential in the laser settings. If the laser pulse duration is less than TRT, the laser energy remains "trapped" within the volume of the irradiated tissue. The strong increase in temperature and the related thermal damage will be located in this region, while the surrounding tissues will undergo very little heating through propagation. If the laser irradiation time is longer, the heat will spread inside the tissue, causing unwanted effects and unpleasant scars (Watanabe et al. 1987).

References

Anderson RR, Parrish JA. Selective photothermolysis: precise microsurgery by selective absorption of pulsed irradiation. Science. 1983;22:524–7.
Apfelberg DB, Maser MR, Lash H. Extended clinical use of the argon laser for cutaneous lesions. Arch Dermatol. 1979;115:719–21.
Apfelberg DB, Maser MR, Lash H, et al. The argon laser for cutaneous lesions. JAMA. 1981;245:2073.

Ara G, Anderson RR, Mandel KG, et al. Irradiation of pigmented melanoma cells with high intensity pulsed radiation generates acoustic waves and kills cells. Lasers Surg Med. 1990;10:52–9.
Boyce S, Alster TS. CO2 laser treatment of epidermal nevi: long-term success. Dermatol Surg. 2002;28:611–4.
Bukvić Mokos Z, Lipozenčić J, Ceović R, et al. Laser therapy of pigmented lesions: pro and contra. Acta Dermatovenerol Croat. 2010;18:185–9.
Castanet J, Ortonne JP. Pigmentary changes in aged and photoaged skin. Arch Dermatol. 1997;133:1296–9.
Dinehart SM, Waner M, Flock S. The copper vapor laser for treatment of cutaneous vascular and pigmented lesions. J Dermatol Surg Oncol. 1993;19:370–5.
Fitzpatrick RE, Goldman MP, Ruiz-Hsparza J. Laser treatment of benign pigmented epidermal lesions usually a 300 nsec pulse and 510 nm wavelength. J Dermatol Surg Oncol. 1993;9:341–7.
Hamilton MM. Laser treatment of pigmented and vascular lesions in the office. Facial Plast Surg. 2004;20:63–9.
Hammes S, Raulin C, Karsai S, et al. Treating papillomatosis intradermal nevi: lasers-yes or no? A prospective study. Hautarzt. 2008;59:101–7.
Kasai K. Picosecond laser treatment for tattoos and benign cutaneous pigmented lesions (Secondary publication). Laser Ther. 2017;26:274–81.
Margolis RJ, Dover JS, Polla LL, et al. Visible action spectrum for melanin-specific selective photothermolysis. Lasers Surg Med. 1989;9(4):389–97.
Patel BC. The krypton yellow-green laser for the treatment of facial vascular and pigmented lesions. Semin Ophthalmol. 1998;13:158–70.
Patil UA, Dhami LD. Overview of lasers. Indian J Plast Surg. 2008;41(Suppl):S101–13.
Polla LL, Margolis RJ, Dover JS, et al. Melanosomes are a primary target of Q-switched ruby laser irradiation in guinea pig skin. J Invest Dermatol. 1987;89:281–6.
Raulin C, Greve B, Grema H. IPL technology: a review. Lasers Surg Med. 2003;32:78–87.
Sardana K. The science, reality, and ethics of treating common acquired melanocytic nevi (moles) with lasers. J Cutan Aesthet Surg. 2013;6:27.
Sebaratnam DF, Lim AC, Lowe PM, et al. Lasers and laser-like devices: part two. Aust J Dermatol. 2014;55:1–14.
Skobelkin OK, Danilin NA, Bogdanov SE, et al. Treatment of pigmented skin lesions with argon laser irradiation. Khirurgiia (Mosk). 1989;91–3.
Stratigos AJ, Dover JS, Arndt KA. Laser treatment of pigmented lesions--2000: how far have we gone? Arch Dermatol. 2000;136:915–21.
Tanzi EL, Lupton JR, Alster TS. Lasers in dermatology: four decades of progress. J Am Acad Dermatol. 2003;49:1–31.
Taylor CR, Anderson RR. Treatment of benign pigmented epidermal lesions by Q- switched ruby laser. Int J Dermatol. 1993;32:908–12.
Vejjabhinanta V, Elsa ML, Patel SS, Patel A, Caperton C, Nouri K. Comparison of short- pulsed and long-pulsed nm lasers in the removal of freckles. Lasers Med Sci. 2010;25:901–6.
Watanabe S, Flotte T, Margolis R. The effects of pulse duration on selective pigmented cell injury by dye lasers. J Invest Dermatol. 1987;88:523.

Type of Lasers Used in This Study

4

As reported in the preface, all the cases presented in this book have been treated with laser or IPL at our "Skin Center" from 2001 onwards and concern Italian patients with skin types that vary between II and III (according to Fitzpatrick's classification scale).

Therefore in this chapter we briefly describe only the types of lasers we have used.

4.1 CO_2 Lasers

The carbon dioxide laser (CO_2 laser) was one of the first gas laser models to be invented (by Kumar Patel at Bell Laboratories in 1964); it is nowadays one of the most widely used in the medical and industrial field.

CO_2 lasers are the most powerful continuous wave lasers available today, and they are also among the most efficient: the ratio between pumping power and laser power can reach 20% (IUPAC n.d.).

This type of laser emits a beam of infrared light whose main wavelength is centered between 9.4 and 10.6 μm. Since CO_2 lasers work in the infrared at a wavelength at which the glass is no longer transparent, special materials are needed for their construction. Generally the mirrors are made of coated silicon or molybdenum, while the lenses and exit windows are of germanium; for high power applications, gold mirrors and windows and zinc selenide lenses are used. Historically, windows and lenses were out of salt (both normal sodium chloride and potassium chloride); while the material was inexpensive, these lenses and windows deteriorated slowly with atmospheric humidity.

The simplest form of CO_2 laser consists of a gas discharge tube (filled with a mixture similar to the one described above) with a totally reflective mirror at one end and an output coupler (usually a semi-reflective mirror of coated zinc selenide)

The contents of this book are partially based on the Italian language edition: "*The Usefulness of Dermoscopy in Laser and IPL Treatments*", Domenico Piccolo, © DEKA M.E.L.A Srl 2012.

© Springer Nature Switzerland AG 2020
D. Piccolo et al., *Quick Guide to Dermoscopy in Laser and IPL Treatments*,
https://doi.org/10.1007/978-3-319-41633-5_4

at the exit end. The reflectivity of the output coupler mirror is usually 5–15%. The laser output, for high power applications, can have a particular coupling (edge-coupled) to reduce the problem of heating the optics.

The CO_2 laser can be designed for powers ranging from a few milliwatts to several hundred kilowatts (kW). It is also very easy to introduce in these lasers a Q-switch device, by means of a rotating mirror or an electro-optical switch, making them capable of generating single power pulses up to one gigawatt (GW).

Since the state transition that gives rise to the laser effect in these devices concerns the vibration-translation bands of a linear triatomic molecule, the rotational structure of the P and R bands can be selected from a tuner element in the cavity of the laser resonator: this element is usually a diffraction grating, because in the infrared band of CO_2 lasers transparent materials generally have rather high losses. By rotating the diffraction grating, a particular rotational line of the vibrational transition can be selected. The finest frequency selection can be obtained using an etalon. Therefore, thanks also to the isotopic substitution, you can select frequencies at will in a range from 880 to 1090 cm^{-1} in a "comb" with intervals of 1 cm^{-1} (30 GHz). However, these "fine-tuned" carbon dioxide lasers are above all of theoretical and research interests.

The sufficiently intense radiations cause the evaporation of the tissue due to the evaporation of the water, with a tissue penetration limited to about 50 μm.

This characteristic, together with the correct management of the pulse, allows to operate with extreme precision in the vaporization of the tissues in successive passages until reaching the clinical end point.

The CO_2 laser is therefore the first choice for laser skin surgery in removing numerous skin lesions such as pigmented melanocytic and non-melanocytic lesions, viral lesions (warts, condyloma acuminatum, molluscum contagiosum), superficial nonmelanoma skin cancers (actinic keratoses, superficial basal cell carcinomas, Bowen's disease), and mucosal lesions (mucoid cysts, genital lesions, leukoplasias, papillomas) (Boyce and Alster 2002; Patil and Dhami 2008) (Fig. 4.1).

4.2 CO_2 Fractional Resurfacing

The latest generation fractional CO_2 laser is an innovative and exclusive surgical laser for aesthetic medicine and dermatology, which is the first to introduce the combined action of the CO_2 laser with radiofrequency (RF) to contrast multiple skin problems. The fractional laser acts by damaging very small fractions of tissue in depth, and leaving the skin undamaged on the surface (Fig. 4.2a–c). The combined action of fractionated CO_2 with RF, known for its principle of heat transfer, has led to a significant stretching of the already evident skin after 5 days and an even more valid resurfacing. The principle is based on the ability of the laser beam to smooth the skin, expand the capillary vessels, and offer a way to spread the RF inside the epidermis. RF restores tone and firmness to the skin, due to its vasoconstricting effect, which significantly reduces healing time and the possible secondary effects of lasers such as redness and edema. RF electromagnetic waves improve the activity of the sodium-potassium pump of the fibroblastic membrane by stimulating the production of elastin and hyaluronic acid. RF has a lifting effect because it contracts collagen to varying degrees of depth.

Fig. 4.1 A laser CO$_2$
device. (Courtesy of
DEKA M.E.L.A. S.r.l.)

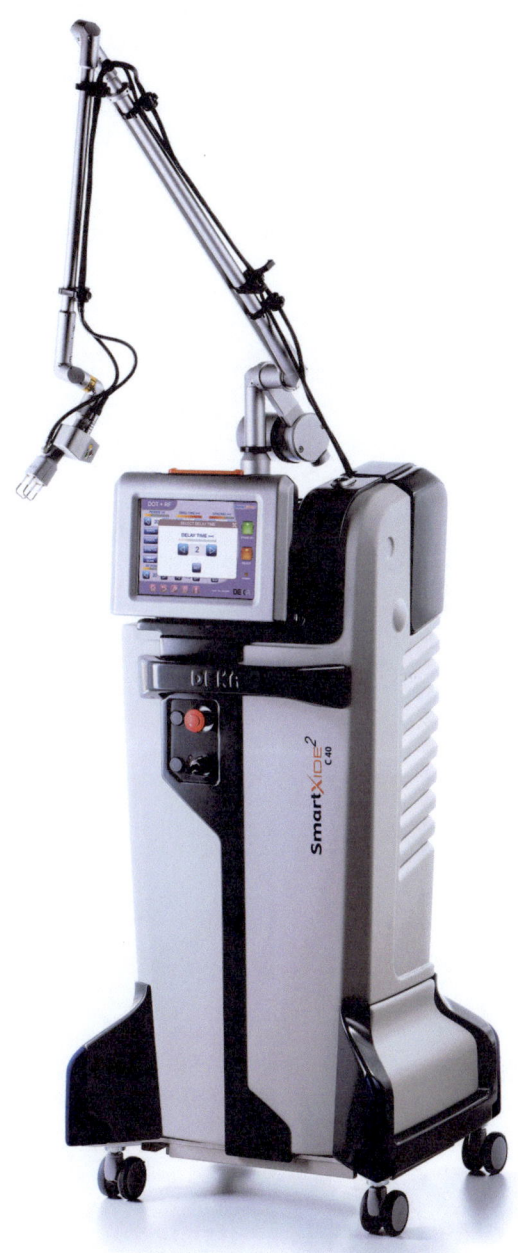

It is an ideal microablative laser for the treatment of photodamage, deep wrinkles of the face, superficial pigmentary disorders, acneic scars, benign pigmented lesions, mini-invasive lifting of the periocular area, firming of the face, and for treating extremely delicate areas such as the face, décolleté, neck, and hands. The treatment lasts about 20 min and an adequate sun protection is recommended for a few weeks after the laser session on the treated area. After an erythema of 3–7 days and variable swelling, the patient resumes his/her common social activities and results will be visible even after only one session after an interval of about a month.

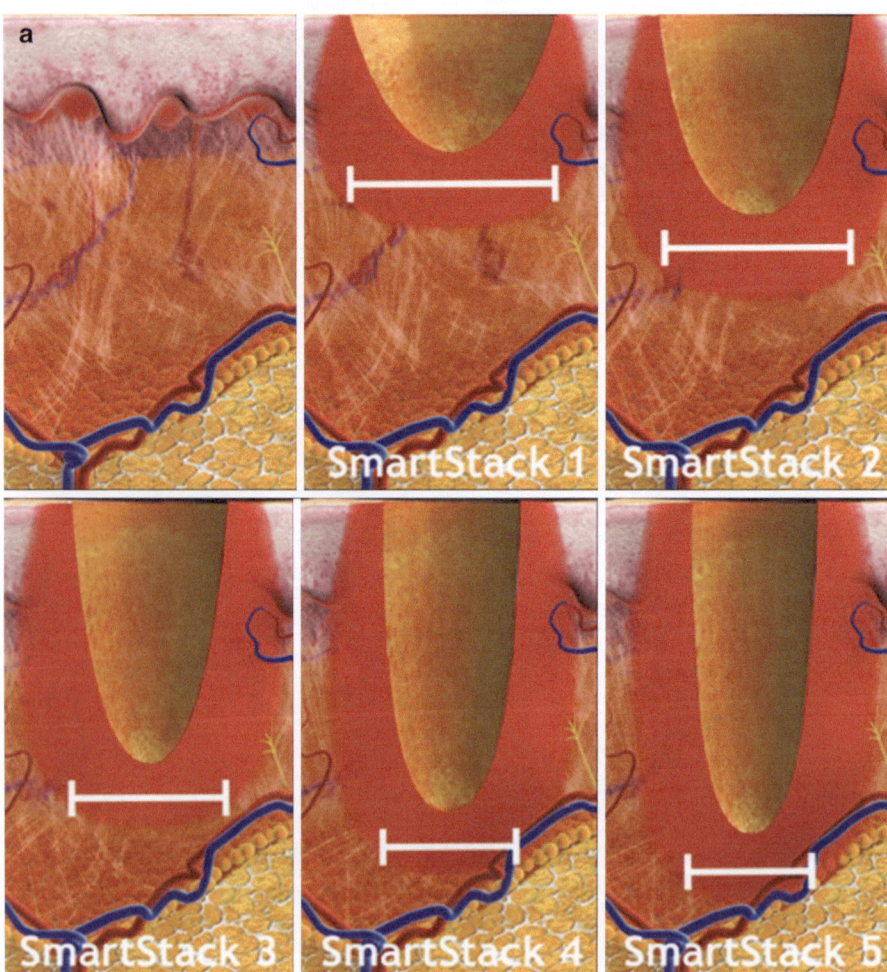

Fig. 4.2 (**a**) Fractional CO_2 and RF and how they work. (**b**) The tip of the handpiece. (**c**) How the tip of the handpiece interacts with the skin. (Courtesy of DEKA M.E.L.A. S.r.l.)

b

c

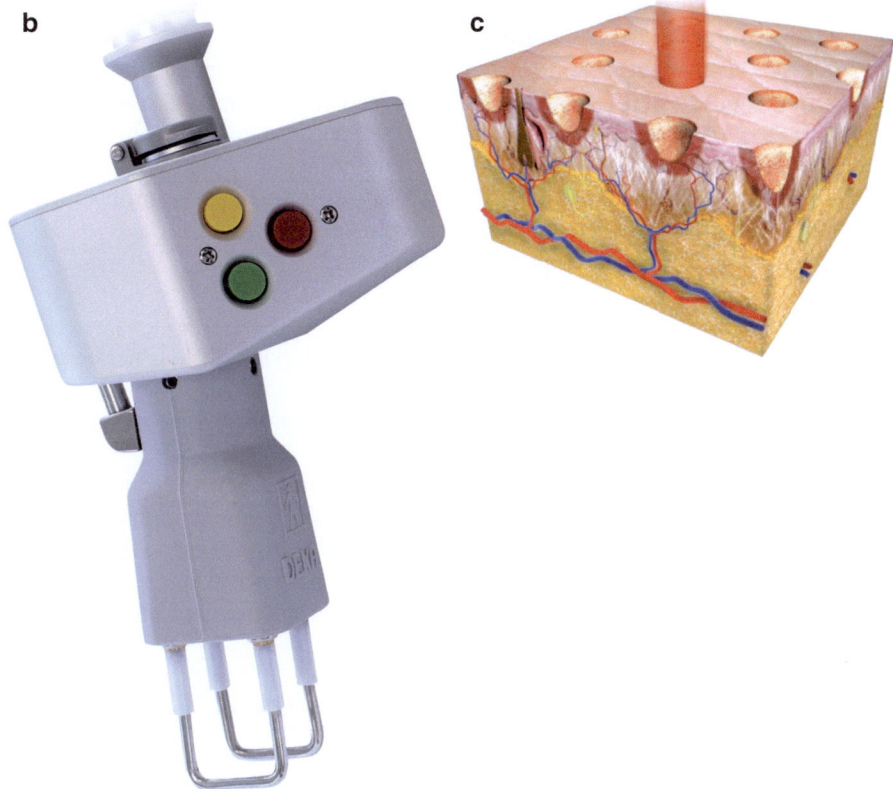

Fig. 4.2 (continued)

4.3 CO_2 Laser and Bipolar Radiofrequency: An Innovative Combination

The simultaneous emission of CO_2 and RF laser waves combines epidermal coagulation for a resurfacing and skin denaturation effect for deeper remodeling.

The development of the CO_2 laser system and the new and more sophisticated operating techniques have led to a considerable increase in the potential applications for surgical lasers, ranging from resurfacing treatments (ablative and fractional) to high precision vaporization of many dermatological lesions, also in very delicate areas such as the eye contour, the external ear, and the mucous and pseudo-mucous areas.

The introduction of innovative CO_2 laser devices, which simultaneously combine fractional CO_2 laser with bipolar RF, guarantees maximum flexibility of operating parameters and perfect adaptation to treatments and skin type.

This combined system generates a special emission from the two sources with specific pulse duration and forms, thus making it highly effective in energy transfer.

Furthermore, the specific shape of the RF electrodes is compatible with the laser emission and allows to operate uniformly on the tissues.

CO_2 lasers induce hyperemia (increase of blood flow to different tissues on the body) in the papillary dermis with a consequent increase in temperature and a reduction in relative tissue impedance. Therefore, the special emission from the handpiece allows a constant passage of the RF current through the blood vessels with an increase in the administered energy: energy transfer is obtained from the surface layers to the deeper layers in a considerably more uniform way.

The device presents several operating parameters:

- *Power* (usually 40, 60, or 80 W).
- *Bipolar RF* (special spacers are inserted which emit bipolar RF to generate selective heating with a deep and localized action on the skin).
- *Number of pulses* (it is usually possible to perform a number of successive pulses in the same place (DOT) between 1 and 5).
- *Time and shape of the impulse* (variable pulse duration, energy, and peak power are provided, allowing users to address any specific treatment condition from different fields of application, from dermatology to gynecology and surgery, and different skin type, to achieve superior results).
- *Distance between DOT* (by selecting both the shape and the size and the spacing of the points based on the treated area).

4.4   Long Pulse 1064 nm Nd:YAG Laser

An Nd:YAG laser is a solid-state laser that uses a neodymium-doped yttrium and aluminum (YAG) crystal as an active laser medium (Nd:Y3Al5O12). Neodymium, vicarious with yttrium, partially replaces it as a trivalent cation in the reticular structure of the YAG. The neodymium content of the mixture is about 1%. The demonstration of the first Nd:YAG laser was carried out, in 1964, at Bell Laboratories (New Jersey, United States).

These lasers normally emit light with a wavelength of 1064 nm, in the infrared, but also have transitions to 940, 1120, 1320, and 1440 nm. The Nd:YAG lasers can work both in continuous and in pulses; in the latter mode they are generally used in Q-switching, i.e., with an optical switch inserted in the resonant cavity which remains closed until the crystal has reached the maximum population inversion, at which time the opening allows the laser to unload a single very high power pulse. In this way it is possible to reach optical powers in output of 20 MW and pulse durations of less than 10 ns.

The Nd:YAG mainly absorbs in the 730–760 and 790–820 nm bands. Therefore, the best excitation is provided by krypton stroboscopic lamps, which emit a lot of light at these frequencies, instead of "normal" xenon lamps.

The amount of dopant neodymium in the material changes according to the use for which it is intended: a laser in continuous wave needs a much weaker doping, while a laser designed to work with pulses needs a lot more doping to have acceptable performances. Nd:YAG rods for continuous wave, weakly doped, are visually recognizable to be less colored, almost white, while those with high doping have a pink-violet color.

Other laser materials that are doped with neodymium are YLF (yttrium and lithium fluoride, 1047 and 1053 nm), YVO4 (yttrium orthovanadate, 1064 nm), and glass. The particular host material is chosen based on the desired mechanical, optical, and thermal characteristics: all these variants are solid-state lasers. Specialized pre-stabilized Nd:YAG lasers (PSL) have been extremely useful for the main beams of gravitational wave interferometers LIGO, VIRGO, GEO600, and TAMA.

Nd:YAG lasers are optically pumped with a stroboscopic lamp or with laser diodes. They are one of the most common types of lasers and have a wide variety of uses in medicine. For instance, ophthalmologists use Nd:YAG lasers in ophthalmic surgery to correct posterior capsular opacification (capsulotomy intervention for secondary cataract): in essence the capsule that supports the artificial crystalline lens with which the natural crystalline has been replaced becomes transparent. Treating patients with glaucoma with narrow angle and open angle closure is also used (if they no longer respond to the pharmacological treatment based on eye drops): in both treatments the intraocular pressure is reduced. Dual frequency Nd:YAG laser (532 nm) versions are also used instead of argon lasers for pan-retinal photocoagulation in patients with diabetic retinopathy.

Also dentists use these lasers for soft tissue surgery of the oral cavity: gingivectomy, periodontal groove drainage, frenulectomy, biopsies, and coagulation of graft donor sites.

In physiotherapy, this laser is used in rehabilitation as a physical therapy for the treatment of scars, whereas in thoracic endoscopy Nd:YAG is used in the endoscopic treatment of benign and malignant tracheal and bronchial stenosis, with or without stent placement.

In dermatology, the Nd:YAG laser is used in progressive hair removal treatments. Furthermore, the special wavelength of the Nd:YAG system and its effective absorption by the hemoglobin makes it possible to reach even the deep blood vessels with a caliber of 1.5–2 mm. The treatment of telangiectasias of the lower limbs presents serious difficulties with respect to facial telangiectasias as the ectatic vessels are located at different depths and present variable hemodynamic characteristics. The effects are immediately visible thanks to the immediate contraction of the vessel accompanied by mild erythema and burning sensation. The latter can be avoided if the laser device has a cooling system (Piccolo et al. 2016).

At the level of the inferior limbs, all laser treatments (mainly for depilation and vascular lesions) have the objective to hit targets located below the epidermis. In these cases it is possible to avoid an excessive increase in the temperature of the epidermis thanks to the cooling system in contact with the skin incorporated in all the handpieces, which prevents the superflex side effects and reduces the sensation of heat.

4.5   Q-Switched (QS) Nd:YAG Laser

First proposed in 1958 by Gordon Gould, and discovered and demonstrated independently in 1961 and 1962 by R.W. Hellwarth and F.J. McClung using Kerr cells as shutters in a ruby laser, Q-switched laser devices represent a technique whereby a laser can produce a pulsed output beam. This technique allows the production with pulses of light with an extremely high peak power (gigawatt), much higher than that produced by the laser itself, if it operated continuously (Nishizawa 2009).

The Q-switched laser system is generally used with two wavelengths: 1064 and 532 nm. This laser represents the gold standard treatment to completely remove tattoos and benign pigmentary disorders because it destroys the pigment without leaving scars or permanent dyschromia.

Unlike dermabrasion and surgical excision, which cause the destruction of tissue in a very generic way, the laser treatment exploits the principle of selective photothermolysis by striking exclusively the pigment contained in the tattoo ink and simultaneously respecting the anatomical integrity of the surrounding skin.

To get these benefits with tattoos, the laser system offers a choice of two wavelengths: 1064 nm for removing blue-black pigment and 532 nm for removing red pigment (Ross et al. 1998).

For the treatment of benign pigmentary disorders, the laser system electively uses the 1064 nm wavelength for the pigment in the deepest dermis and the wavelength of 532 nm to remove a more superficial pigment.

To contain the pulse time within the TRT of both the tattoo pigment and melanin, laser systems allow emissions of only nano-second pulses (ns). With this pulse mode, three different effects on the pigment are obtained (Fig. 4.3).

The photomechanical effect induces a rapid fragmentation of the pigment due to the rapid expansion of the heat. In the case of benign pigmentary pathologies, this rapid expansion induces the lysis of the melanocytic cell which gives rise to the elimination of the deepest pigment through the phagocytes, while the most superficial pigment is eliminated transepidermically (Kilmer and Garden 2000) (Fig. 4.4).

Furthermore, it is possible to create a photochemical effect on the tattoo, which induces pyrolytic alterations in the pigment by varying its optical characteristics and thus making it less visible. A dermis fibrosis process can be subsequently observed around the fragmented ink particles, thus leading to their optical obscuration.

4.6   Dye Lasers

Dye lasers were discovered independently by P. P. Sorokin and F. P. Schäfer (and colleagues) in 1966 (Magyar 1974).

The dye laser is a type of selective laser for the treatment of all red skin aestheticism, as it acts exclusively on that type of pigment. A dye laser is a laser that uses an organic dye as a laser medium, usually as a liquid solution. Compared to gases and most solid-state laser means, a dye can usually be used for a much wider range

Fig. 4.3 QS laser:
schematic explanation.
(Courtesy of DEKA
M.E.L.A. S.r.l.)

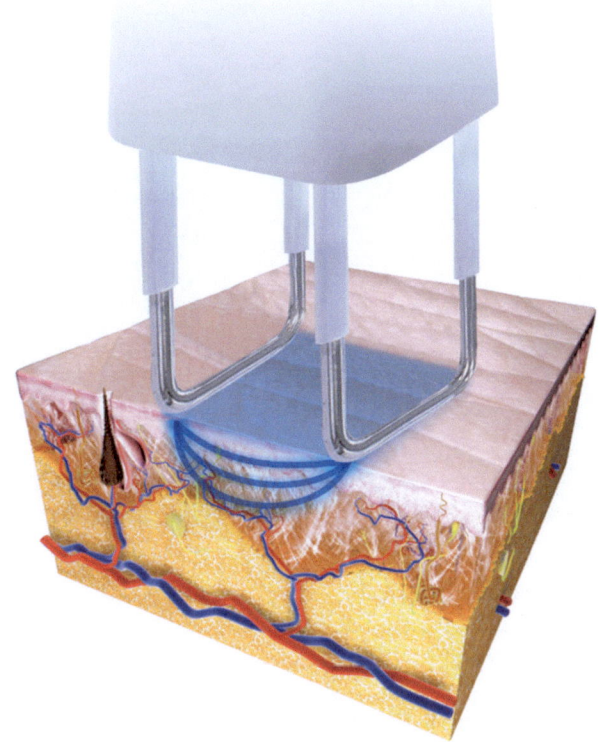

of wavelengths, often from 50 to 100 nm or more. The treatment is almost painless and the results are visible after a couple of months (Faurschou et al. 2009).

Thanks to its selectivity it allows to treat all the red skin aestheticisms, and is indicated in particular for the treatment of:

- Capillaries (telangiectasias)
- Couperose and rosacea
- Angiomas (flat, stellar, ruby)
- Scars during inflammation
- Erythrosis
- Telangiectatic matting
- Poikiloderma of Civatte (a sort of couperose on the neck)
- Stretch marks in the inflammatory phase

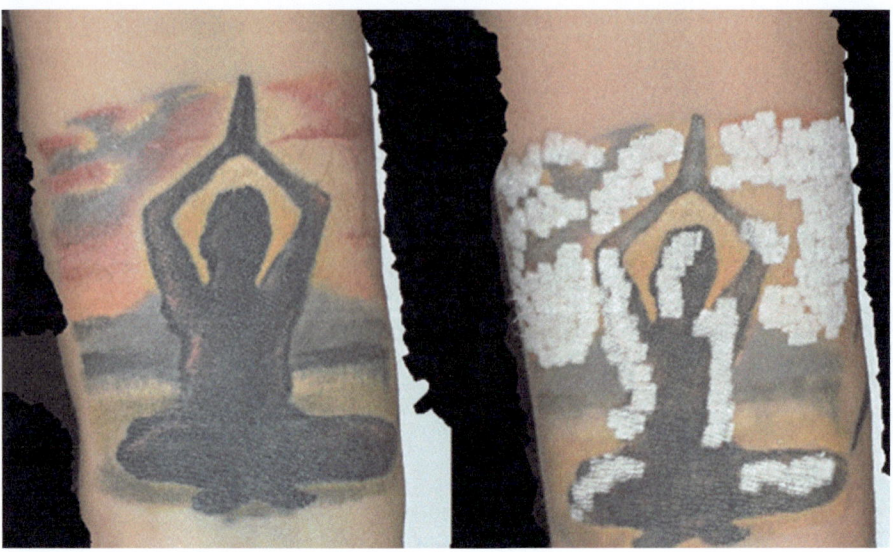

Fig. 4.4 QS laser: example of application in tattoo removal. (Courtesy of Dr. Domenico Piccolo, Skin Center Avezzano, Italy)

References

Boyce S, Alster TS. CO2 laser treatment of epidermal nevi: long-term success. Dermatol Surg. 2002;28:611–4.

Faurschou A, Togsverd-Bo K, Zachariae C, et al. Pulsed dye laser vs. intense pulsed light for port-wine stains: a randomized side-by-side trial with blinded response evaluation. Br J Dermatol. 2009;160:359–64.

IUPAC. Gold Book, carbon dioxide laser (CO2 laser). n.d. http://goldbook.iupac.org/.

Kilmer SL, Garden JM. Laser treatment of pigmented lesions and tattoos. Semin Cutan Med Surg. 2000;19(4):232–44.

Magyar G. Dye lasers--a classified bibliography 1966-1972. Appl Opt. 1974;13(1):25–45.

Nishizawa J. Extension of frequencies from maser to laser. How the laser evolved and was extended to terahertz during my research life: a personal review. Proc Jpn Acad Ser B Phys Biol Sci. 2009;85(10):454–65.

Patil UA, Dhami LD. Overview of lasers. Indian J Plast Surg. 2008;41(Suppl):S101–13.

Piccolo D, Crisman G, Kostaki D, et al. Rhodamine intense pulsed light versus conventional intense pulsed light for facial telangiectasias. J Cosmet Laser Ther. 2016;18(2):80–5. https://doi.org/10.3109/14764172.2015.1114641.

Ross V, Naseef G, Lin G, et al. Comparison of responses of tattoos to picosecond and nanosecond Q-switched neodymium: YAG lasers. Arch Dermatol. 1998;134(2):167–71.

Noncoherent Light Sources: IPL and PDT Basic Principles

5

Intense pulsed light (IPL) is a device that emits polychromatic, noncoherent light usually in the 400–1200 nm range. With the aid of convertible "cutoff" filters that guarantee the desired wavelength, associated with a wide spectrum of possible combinations of pulse duration, pulse sequences, pulse delay time, and fluences, IPL devices offer an alternative therapeutic option for several dermatologic conditions (Piccolo 2012). Pigmentary disorders, especially solar lentigines and diffuse dyschromia (Moreno Arias and Ferrando 2001; Kawada et al. 2002; Raulin et al. 2003), as well as hair removal and vascular lesions can be effectively and safely treated with IPL (Babilas et al. 2007; Piccolo et al. 2016) (Fig. 5.1).

To avoid energy loss, before each treatment it is necessary to apply a thin layer of transparent gel (such as that used for ultrasound scans) between the skin and the handpiece.

Thanks to the skin cooling device built into the handpiece of some IPL devices (like the one used in both our Skin Center), patients seem to suffer less pain even if the pain depends on the area treated and the type of treatment (Piccolo et al. 2014).

Intervals between sessions may vary from 2 to 3 weeks after vascular treatment and photorejuvenation, and up to 1–2 months after hair removal. The number of applications depends on the pathology or imperfection to be treated. Random clinical studies of IPL have demonstrated a gradual and significant improvement in multiple clinical conditions such as facial telangiectasis, spider nevi, hyperchromia, melasma, hypertrichosis, and wrinkles.

Selective photothermolysis (absorption of melanin in the hair) causes thermal destruction of the follicle without damaging the surrounding tissues (Anderson and Parrish 1983). The pulsed light emissions stimulate the fibroblasts in a noninvasive manner, inducing the production of new collagen fibers, and thus easing wrinkles.

Thanks to selective photothermolysis and the choice of different filters, this device can also destroy the melanin in the deeper layers of the epidermis, reducing

The contents of this book are partially based on the Italian language edition: "*The Usefulness of Dermoscopy in Laser and IPL Treatments*", Domenico Piccolo, © DEKA M.E.L.A Srl 2012.

© Springer Nature Switzerland AG 2020

D. Piccolo et al., *Quick Guide to Dermoscopy in Laser and IPL Treatments*,
https://doi.org/10.1007/978-3-319-41633-5_5

Fig. 5.1 Simplified differences between IPL and laser in the emission of the light beam. (Courtesy of DEKA M.E.L.A. S.r.l.)

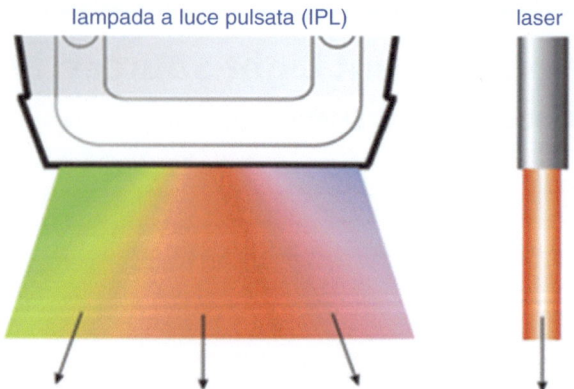

hyperchromia and improving skin texture. Furthermore, IPL mechanism of action in treating superficial benign pigmented lesions is thought to be the result of rapid differentiation of keratinocytes induced by thermal heating. This process leads to an upward transfer of melanosomes along with necrotic keratinocytes, resulting in their elimination as the crusts are removed from the skin surface (Yamashita et al. 2006) (Fig. 5.2a–c).

According to the literature, even though its use and effectiveness are strongly related to the operator's experience, IPL demonstrates high efficacy rates, minimal discomfort (mild burning sensation and slight erythema are the most common side effects, which spontaneously resolve within 24–96 h), rapid treatment and recovery times, and excellent cosmetic and therapeutic outcomes in a wide range of dermatological disease, including NMSCs (Piccolo and Kostaki 2018).

Thus, IPL is such a versatile tool, which is relatively painless, which grants rapid treatment and recovery times and excellent cosmetic outcomes, and represents an effective and precious ally in dermatology practice.

5.1   Photodynamic Therapy (PDT)

Photodynamic therapy is a therapeutic option for nonmelanoma skin cancers (NMSCs) and precancerous conditions such as actinic keratoses (AKs), which involves the sequential use of a photosensitizing product, locally administered, and a light source suitable for activating it. In the presence of oxygen-containing tissues, a photodynamic reaction occurs with the production of oxygen-free radicals and the consequent cell death. The photosensitizer for cutaneous PDT must be a nontoxic molecule for humans, small to penetrate through the skin, and able to select between healthy cells and diseased or tumor cells. The 5-aminolevulinic acid (5-ALA) has been shown to possess these characteristics and is therefore the most used photosensitizer molecule in PDT (Bernstein et al. 1990; Downs et al. 2009).

The light represents the energy needed to activate the drug, in this case Protoporphyrin IX (PpIX). The light to be administered must not have a biological effect, such as in LASER treatments, where it is the light itself that destroys the cells. It is only a matter of triggering a photochemical reaction and activating PpIX. To check if 5-ALA has penetrated and if it has been transformed into PpIX

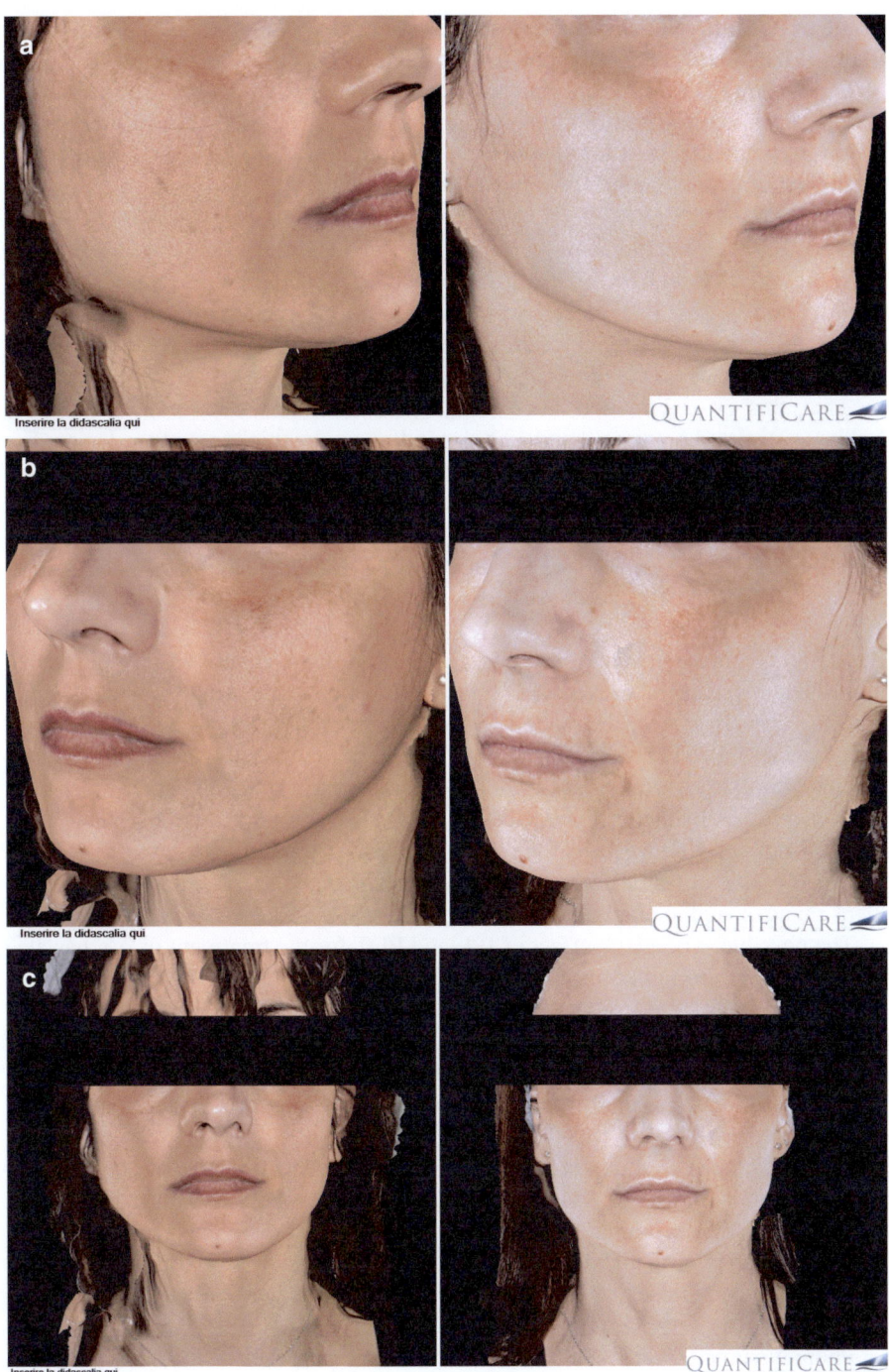

Fig. 5.2 (**a–c**) Comparison of the clinical presentation of facial hyperpigmentations in a young woman before and after four IPL sessions. An excellent outcome has been reached. (Courtesy of Dr. Domenico Piccolo, Skin Center Avezzano, Italy)

inside tumor cells, the clinician illuminates the area with a Wood light lamp (black light): if a dark red color will appear, then the reaction has occurred.

Before any PDT treatment, it is important that the patient suspends the intake of potentially photosensitizing drugs. Moreover, it is often necessary to prepare the lesions to be treated in order to increase the absorption of 5-ALA (e.g., if the lesion is covered by a crust, it must be removed, even with the CO_2 laser, which in this case is a great option).

5-ALA is an unstable acid, so it must be prepared just before application or at most the day before. The 5–20% 5-ALA cream is then applied to the lesions. An occlusive dressing is then placed over a layer of polystyrene to improve the absorption of the photosensitizer in the lesion to be treated also because the light input could partially deactivate the 5-ALA.

After this procedure it is necessary to wait for the complete penetration of 5-ALA, estimated between 3 and 12 h depending on the thickness of the lesion. For inflammatory diseases and photorejuvenation, the application time drops to 1 h and 30 min (Kim et al. 2005; Moloney and Collins 2007; Kohl et al. 2017).

5.2   Interactions Between IPL and PDT

By studying photorejuvenation process, several authors described an unexpected high clearance rate of related AKs presented by patients. Ruiz-Rodriguez et al. (2002) achieved an AKs clearance rate of 87% at 3-month follow-up, with the combined use of ALA-PDT and IPL for the treatment of AK and photodamage in 17 patients. Similarly, Avram and Goldman (2004) also treated 17 patients with photodamage and AK using an IPL device for ALA-PDT and obtained a 69% reduction of AK with an IPL treatment. In both studies, photorejuvenation effects were observed on the areas of the treated skin, in terms of skin structure, wrinkles, pigment changes, and telangiectasias.

The possible synergistic effect of IPL and PDT for the treatment of AK has also been addressed in numerous comparative studies. Gold et al. (2006) conducted a comparative split-face study using ALA-IPL vs. IPL alone for photorejuvenation and showed an increase in the clearance rate of AK with a short contact (30–60 min) ALA-PDT and IPL vs. IPL alone (78% versus 53.6%) after three sessions with an interval of 1 month. Furthermore, an improvement was observed in several photoaging parameters.

Thanks to its large spot size, IPL allows the treatment of multiple lesions in different anatomical areas in a significantly shorter time. With a suitable filter and a specific program, it is possible to use IPL as a light source to activate 5-aminolevulinic acid. Triggered photodynamic therapy is able to treat all superficial epithelial tumors such as actinic keratoses and basal cell carcinomas (Hasegawa et al. 2010; Haddad et al. 2011).

Photodynamic therapy is also used for aesthetic purposes or for dermatological diseases. In the first case, various skin imperfections can be treated such as wrinkles, acne scars, and hair removal. Inflammatory diseases of dermatological interest

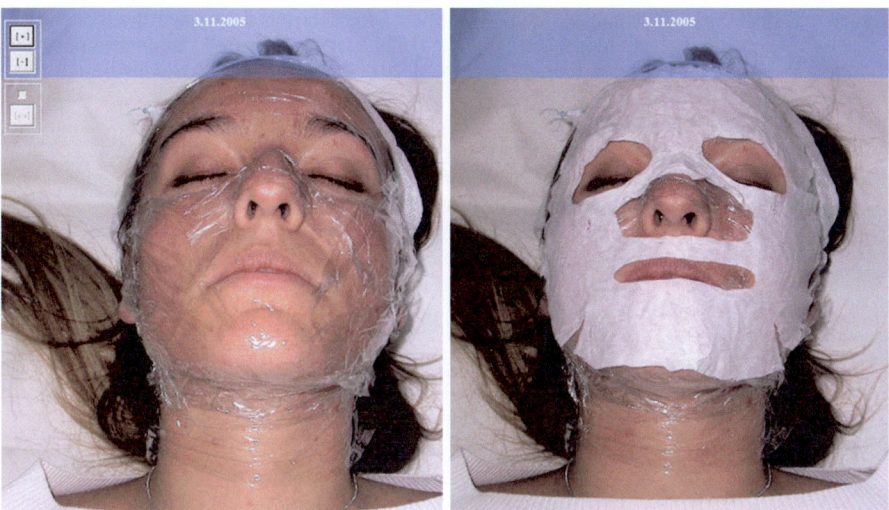

Fig. 5.3 A patient prepared for a PDT with IPL session. (Courtesy of Dr. Domenico Piccolo, Skin Center Avezzano, Italy)

that can be treated with PDT include acne and alopecia areata. Furthermore, IPL devices have proven effective in the simultaneous treatment of apparent sun-damaged skin and AK (Piccolo and Kostaki 2018) (Fig. 5.3). Disadvantages of the IPL-PDT are related to the possible inconsistency of the light spectrum emitted, in particular in older IPL devices containing a small bank of capacitors (Haddad et al. 2009). Moreover, unwanted hair reduction may occur in the treated area.

References

Anderson RR, Parrish JA. Selective photothermolysis: precise microsurgery by selective absorption of pulsed irradiation. Science. 1983;22:524–7.

Avram DK, Goldman MP. Effectiveness and safety of ALA-IPL in treating actinic keratoses and photodamage. J Drugs Dermatol. 2004;3:S36–9.

Babilas P, Knobler R, Hummel S, et al. Variable pulsed light is less painful than light- emitting diodes for topical photodynamic therapy of actinic keratosis: a prospective randomized controlled trial. Br J Dermatol. 2007;157:111–7.

Bernstein EF, Thomas GF, Smith PD, et al. Response of black and white guinea pig skin to photodynamic treatment using 514-nm light and dihematoporphyrin ether. Arch Dermatol. 1990;126:1303–7.

Downs AM, Bower CB, Oliver DA, et al. Methyl aminolaevulinate-photodynamic therapy for actinic keratoses, squamous cell carcinoma in situ and superficial basal cell carcinoma employing a square wave intense pulsed light device for photoactivation. Br J Dermatol. 2009;161:189–90.

Gold MH, Bradshaw VL, Boring MM, et al. Split-face comparison of photodynamic therapy with 5-aminolevulinic acid and intense pulsed light versus intense pulsed light alone for photodamage. Dermatol Surg. 2006;32:795–801.

Haddad A, Santos ID, Gragnani A, et al. The effect of increasing fluence on the treatment of actinic keratosis and photodamage by photodynamic therapy with 5- aminolevulinic acid and intense pulsed light. Photomed Laser Surg. 2011;29(6):427–32. https://doi.org/10.1089/pho.2009.2733.

Hasegawa T, Suga Y, Mizuno Y, et al. Efficacy of photodynamic therapy with topical 5- aminolevulinic acid using intense pulsed light for Bowen's disease. J Dermatol. 2010;37:623–8.

Kawada A, Shiraishi H, Asai M, et al. Clinical improvement of solar lentigines and ephelides with an intense pulsed light source. Dermatol Surg. 2002;28:504–8.

Kim HS, Yoo JY, Cho KH, et al. Topical photodynamic therapy using intense pulsed light for treatment of actinic keratosis: clinical and histopathologic evaluation. Dermatol Surg. 2005;31:33–6.

Kohl E, Popp C, Zeman F, et al. Photodynamic therapy using intense pulsed light for treating actinic keratoses and photoaged skin of the dorsal hands: a randomized placebo-controlled study. Br J Dermatol. 2017;176:352–62.

Moloney FJ, Collins P. Randomized, double-blind, prospective study to compare topical 5-aminolaevulinic acid methylester with topical 5-aminolaevulinic acid photodynamic therapy for extensive scalp actinic keratosis. Br J Dermatol. 2007;157:87–91.

Moreno Arias GA, Ferrando J. Intense Pulsed Light for Melanocytic Lesions. Dermatol Surg. 2001;27(4):397–400.

Piccolo D. The usefulness of dermoscopy in laser and intense pulsed light treatments. Florence: Remo Sandron Edition; 2012.

Piccolo D, Kostaki D. Photodynamic therapy activated by intense pulsed light in the treatment of non-melanoma skin cancer. Biomedicine. 2018;6(1):E18.

Piccolo D, Di Marcantonio D, Crisman G, et al. Unconventional use of intense pulsed light. Biomed Res Int. 2014;2014:618206.

Piccolo D, Crisman G, Kostaki D, et al. Rhodamine intense pulsed light versus conventional pulsed light for facial teleangiectasias. J Cosmet Laser Ther. 2016;18(2):80–5.

Raulin C, Greve B, Hortensia Grema. IPL technology: A review. Lasers Surg Med. 2003;32(2):78–87.

Ruiz-Rodriguez R, Sanz-Sánchez T, Córdoba S. Photodynamic photorejuvenation. Dermatol Surg. 2002;28:742–4.

Yamashita T, Negishi K, Hariya T, et al. Intense Pulsed Light Therapy for Superficial Pigmented Lesions Evaluated by Reflectance-Mode Confocal Microscopy and Optical Coherence Tomography. J Investig Dermatol. 2006;126(10):2281–86.

Dermoscopy Applied to Lasers and IPL Treatments: Melanocytic Nevi

6

The use of lasers to treat melanocytic nevi has been subject to debate because of concerns about their possible malignant transformation (Stratigos et al. 2000; Sardana 2013). In the last few years, it has become relatively clear that laser irradiation is unlikely to increase malignant potential. To date, surgical excision is the standard approach in the removal of these lesions since it allows a histopathologic examination and then the exclusion of cellular atypia. However, the presence of some melanocytic nevi in positions sensitive from the aesthetic or functional point of view, in which surgical removal is difficult to obtain or which will probably leave a noticeable scar, may limit this procedure. Therefore, in these cases laser treatment is preferably applied. To date, different types of laser for melanocytic nevi have been proposed with variable clinical outcomes (Bray et al. 2016; Arora et al. 2015; Hammes et al. 2008; Ohmaru et al. 2011; Zeng et al. 2016).

Based on the available evidence (Omi and Numano 2014; Köse 2018; Angermair et al. 2015), in our daily practice we use laser treatment for the removal of intradermal nevi. Intradermal nevi are common acquired melanocytic nevi that can be clinically presented as papules, plaques, or nodules with a pedunculated, papillomatous (Unna nevus), or smooth (Miescher nevus) surface. These lesions can be aesthetically annoying or can be traumatized by jewelry and clothing, and therefore their removal is a frequent requirement in dermatological practice.

We believe that from an aesthetic point of view, the ultra-pulsed CO_2 laser device is the best option for these lesions, due to the ease of resection, less bleeding, minimal post-treatment edema and pain, and inconspicuous scars when applied correctly.

The contents of this book are partially based on the Italian language edition: "*The Usefulness of Dermoscopy in Laser and IPL Treatments*", Domenico Piccolo, © DEKA M.E.L.A Srl 2012.

© Springer Nature Switzerland AG 2020
D. Piccolo et al., *Quick Guide to Dermoscopy in Laser and IPL Treatments*,
https://doi.org/10.1007/978-3-319-41633-5_6

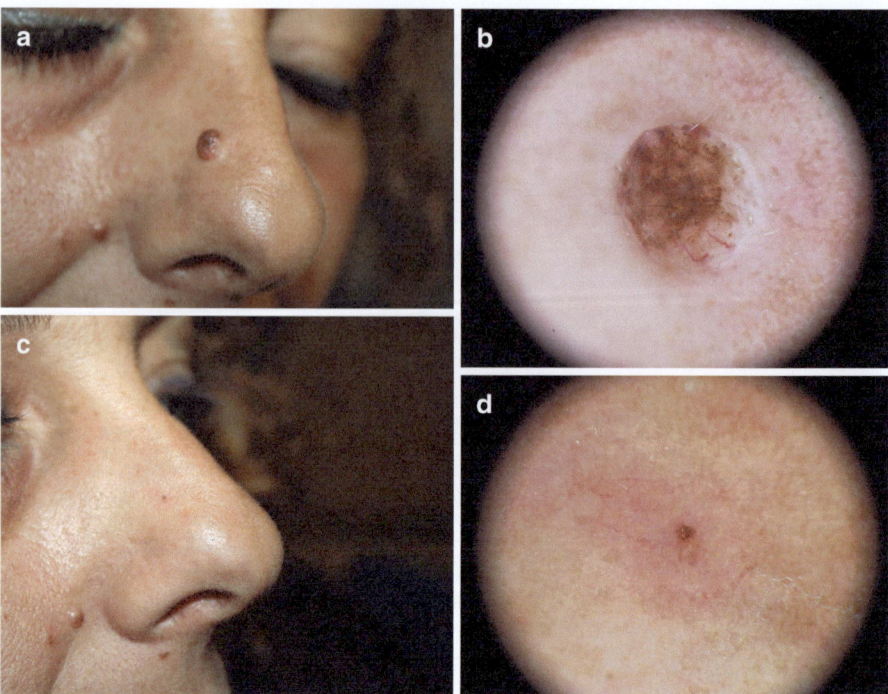

Fig. 6.1 (**a**) Clinical picture of a papillomatous nevus on the wing of the nose in a woman before any treatment. (**b**) Dermoscopic image of the lesion. (**c**) Clinical image after laser CO_2 excision. (**d**) Dermoscopic exam highlights a complete clearance of the pigmented lesion. (Courtesy of Dr. Domenico Piccolo, Skin Center Avezzano, Italy)

6.1   The Validity of Dermoscopy in the Treatment of Melanocytic Nevi

Dermoscopy is essential for laser treatment management. Before any laser treatment (such as a CO_2 laser excision), dermoscopy should be performed for both diagnostic and medical-legal purposes (Figs. 6.1a, b, 6.2a, b, 6.3a, b, 6.4a, b, 6.5a, b, and 6.6a, b). The acquired dermoscopic images before treatment can demonstrate the feasibility of the treatment itself. Indeed, the presence of a globular or cobblestone pattern and/or the presence of papillomatous structures demonstrates the maturation of the lesion and thus the feasibility of using laser even in the absence of a histopathological examination (Argenziano et al. 2003). Dermoscopy is also important for understanding the levels of ablation during treatment and thus preventing scarring, and the dermoscopic examination immediately after the treatment can be used to determine the absence or presence of nevus cell residues and/or thermal damage. Furthermore, dermoscopy after some time (4-week average follow-up) is useful for early detection of nevus cell residues and eventually to decide to proceed with a new laser session. Otherwise, dermoscopic examination of a lesion perfectly removed with the CO_2 laser usually reveals the persistence of erythema and an increase in the vascular pattern that fade over time (Figs. 6.1c, d, 6.2c, d, 6.3c, d, 6.4c, d, 6.5c, d, and 6.6c, d).

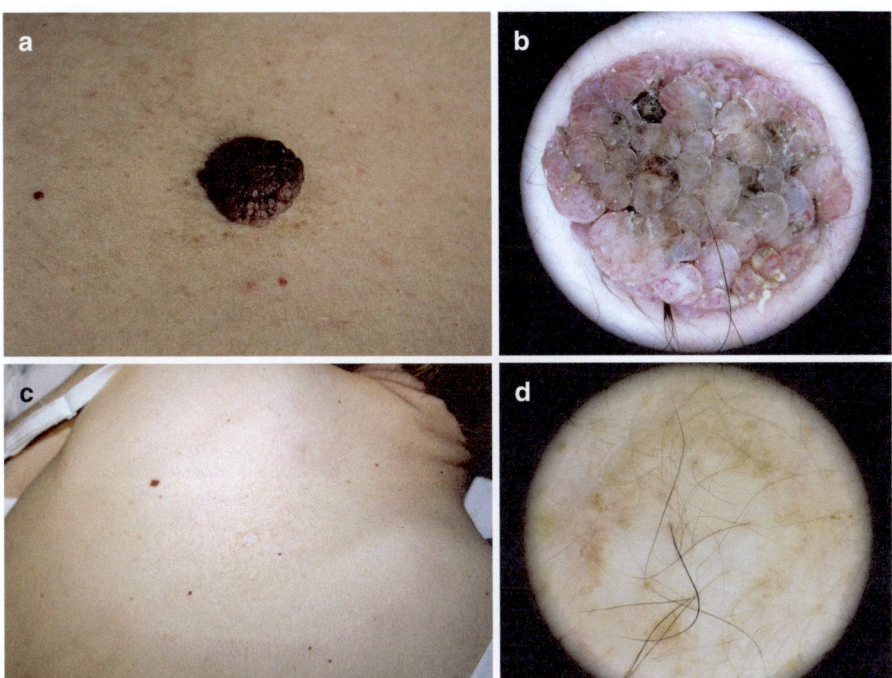

Fig. 6.2 (**a**) Clinical picture of a papillomatous nevus on the back in a boy before any treatment. (**b**) Dermoscopic image of the lesion. (**c**) Clinical image after laser CO_2 excision. (**d**) Dermoscopic exam highlights a complete clearance of the pigmented lesion. (Courtesy of Dr. Domenico Piccolo, Skin Center Avezzano, Italy)

Modern software for pictures analysis helped both clinicians and patients to observe and evaluate the achieved outcome with the possibility of a direct comparison of clinical images taken before any treatment and at the final follow-up visit (Fig. 6.6e, f).

Laser or IPL therapy should not be considered as a treatment option for melanocytic nevi. However, accidental exposure of these lesions to light systems, particularly during hair removal procedures, has been reported so far. In a nevus lying in the field of laser treatment, the increased number of melanocytes and melanin may become an accidental target for light hair removal devices resulting in clinical, dermoscopic, and histopathologic changes (Sillard et al. 2013; Garrido-Ríos et al. 2013; Álvarez-Garrido et al. 2016; Pampín Franco et al. 2016) (Fig. 6.7a–c).

Clinical changes consist of inflammation, oozing, swelling, and crust formation. The dermoscopic images immediately after IPL treatment show modifications

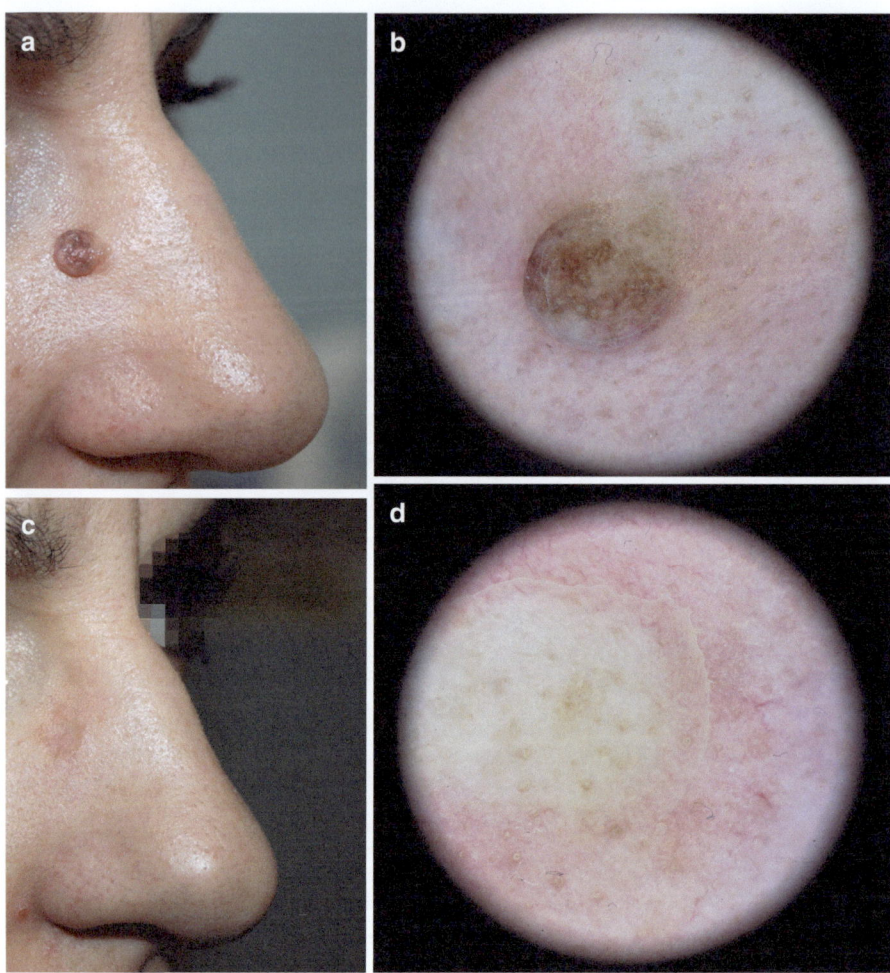

Fig. 6.3 (**a**) Clinical picture of a papillomatous nevus on the wing of the nose in a woman before any treatment. (**b**) Dermoscopic image of the lesion. (**c**) Clinical image after laser CO_2 excision. (**d**) Dermoscopic exam highlights a complete clearance of the pigmented lesion. (Courtesy of Dr. Domenico Piccolo, Skin Center Avezzano, Italy)

similar to those seen after UV exposure with an increase in pigmentation, reinforcement of the pigment network, and the presence of inflammation. Other modifications reported in the literature include milky red veil, gray blue dots as well as blue–grayish and whitish areas (Hammes et al. 2008; Sillard et al. 2013; Pampín Franco et al. 2016). These changes may be completely reversible few months after treatment. Dermoscopic evaluation can document the complete disappearance of

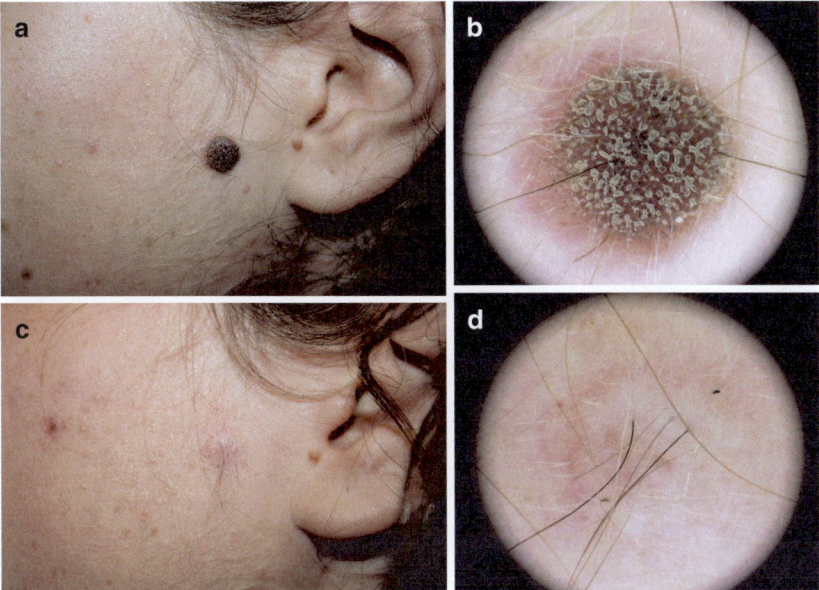

Fig. 6.4 (**a**) Clinical picture of a papillomatous nevus on the cheek of a woman before any treatment. (**b**) Dermoscopy image of the lesion. (**c**) Clinical image after laser CO_2 excision. (**d**) Dermoscopic exam highlights a complete clearance of the pigmented lesion. (Courtesy of Dr. Domenico Piccolo, Skin Center Avezzano, Italy)

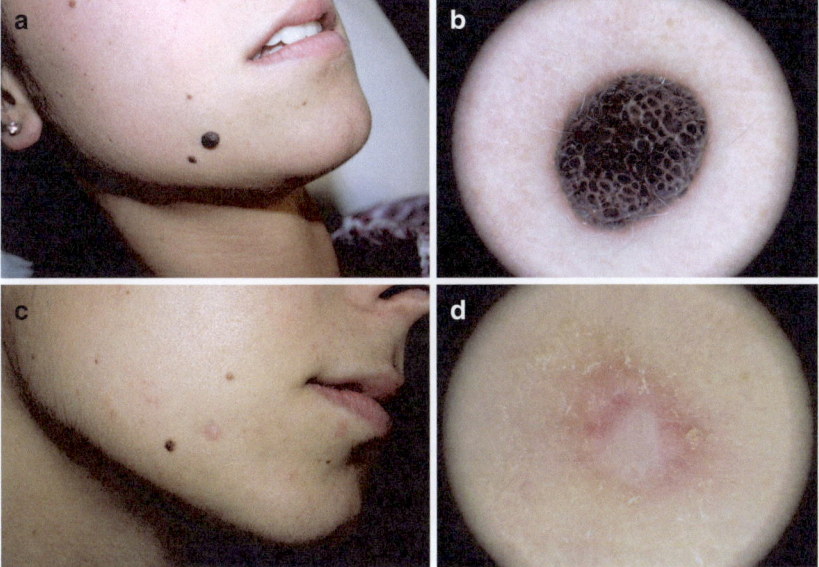

Fig. 6.5 (**a**) Clinical picture of a papillomatous nevus sited on the cheek of a young woman. (**b**) Dermoscopy image of the lesion. (**c**) Clinical image after a laser CO_2 session. (**d**) Dermoscopic exam highlights a complete clearance of the pigmented lesion. (Courtesy of Dr. Domenico Piccolo, Skin Center Avezzano, Italy)

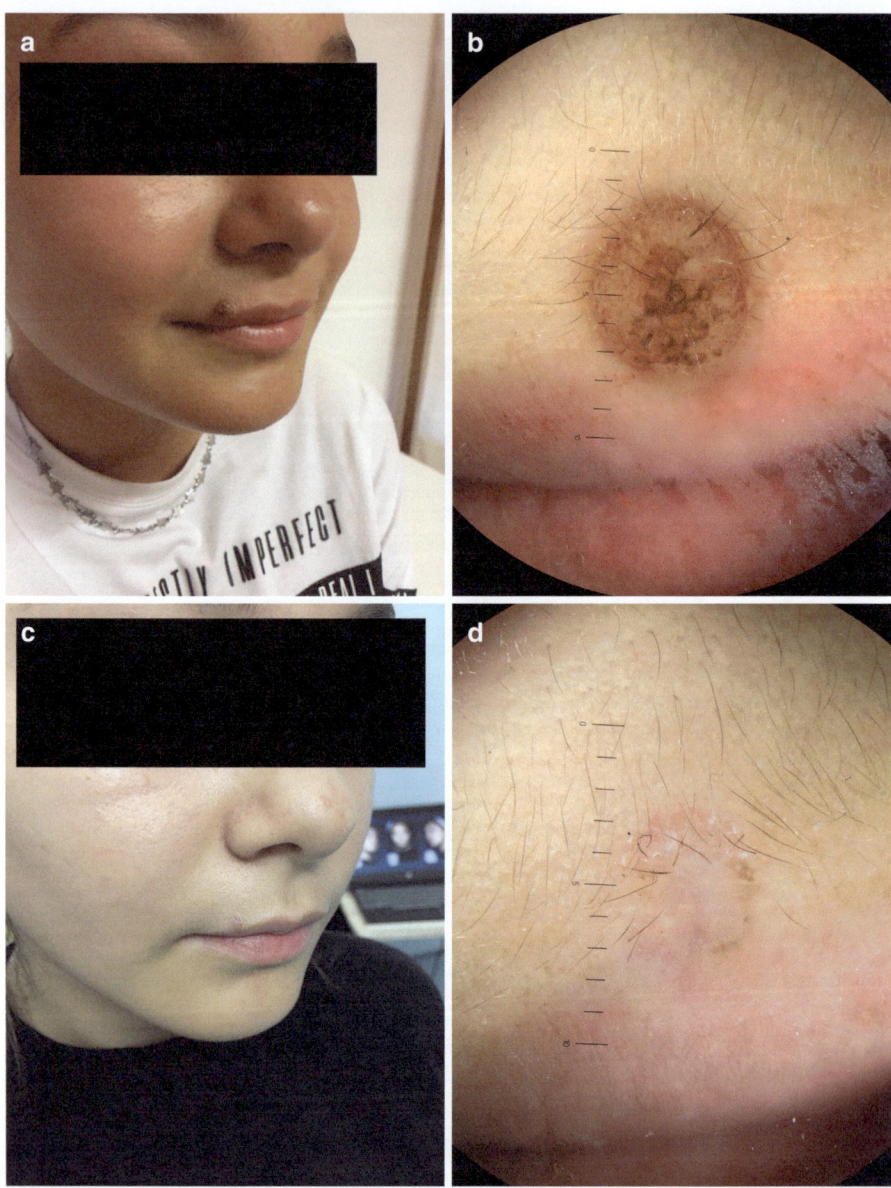

Fig. 6.6 (**a**) Papillomatous dermal nevus on the upper lip of a girl. (**b**) Dermoscopic exam confirming the clinical diagnosis. (**c**) Clinical picture after removal with a single CO_2 laser session. (**d**) Dermoscopic exam highlights the complete removal of the lesion. (**e, f**) Software automatic comparison before and after treatment: this option offers to both the clinician and patient the possibility to observe and evaluate the achieved outcome. An excellent outcome, in this particular case. (Courtesy of Dr. Domenico Piccolo, Skin Center Avezzano, Italy)

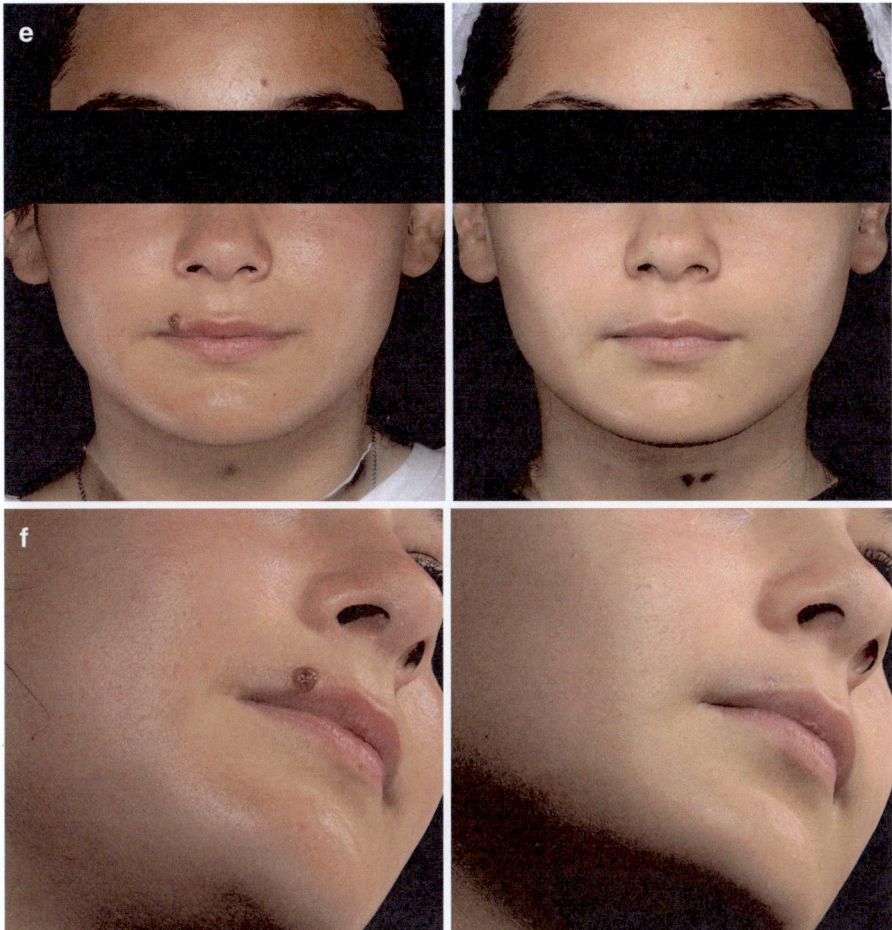

Fig. 6.6 (continued)

the modifications and a return to the pretreatment condition. However, in some cases, long-standing changes may occur, thus leading to a complete or partial destruction of the nevus treated. Dermoscopy can detect such regressive phenomena with the presence of pepper-like structures. Zalaudek et al. (2004) analyzed a series of 158 melanocytic nevi with dermoscopic features of regression (blue-white structures). On histological examination, the lesions showing a regression in more than 50% of their surface presented atrophy of the epidermal ridges and rare residual melanocytes on the basal layer, with numerous melanophages and ectatic vessels in the superficial dermis. A complete dermoscopic regression of a nevus has been reported once with IPL (Martın et al. 2012).

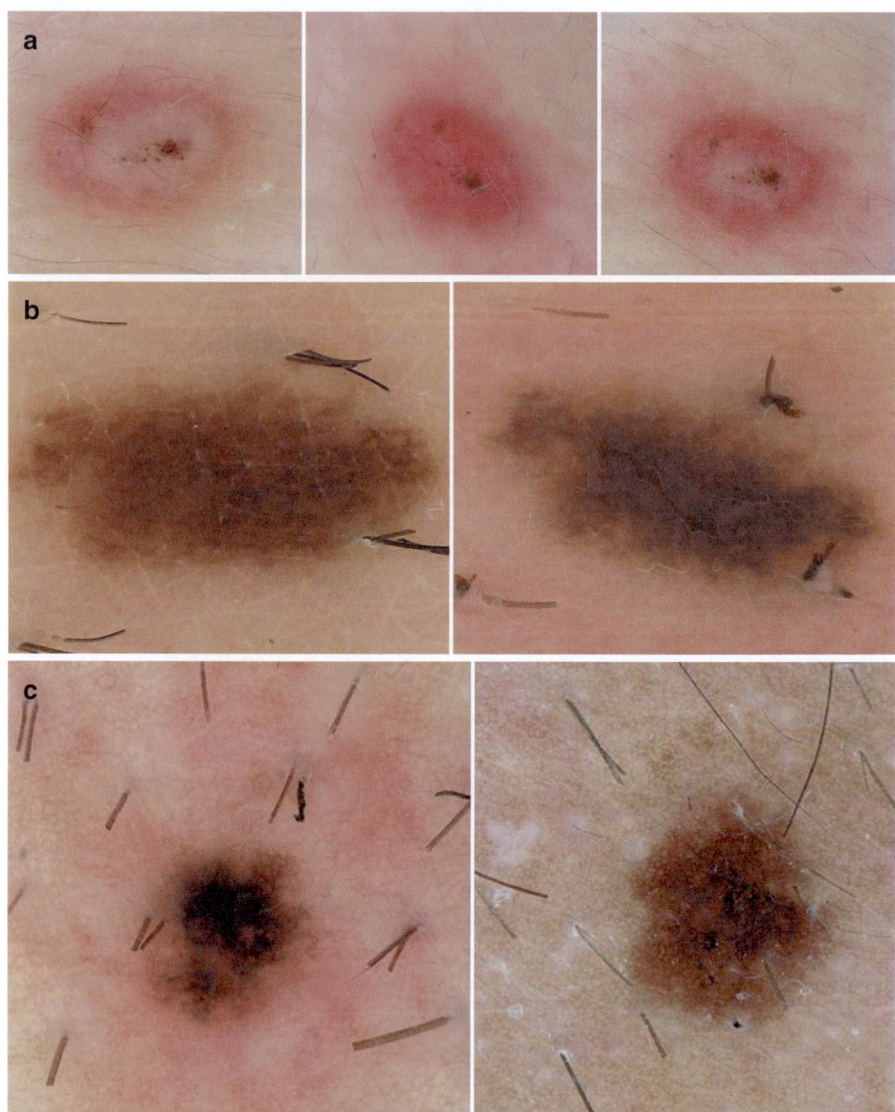

Fig. 6.7 (**a**) Melanocytic nevi should not be treated with IPL. However, papillomatous dermal nevi only present inflammation immediately after the treatment and clears up completely 2 months after treatment. (**b**) Clark nevi (sporadically hit) show typical sun-damaged modifications such as increase of pigmentation, thickness of pigment network, and presence of inflammation. (**c**) Usually, these phenomena completely regress 1–2 months after the treatment as shown in this case. (Courtesy of Dr. Domenico Piccolo, Skin Center Avezzano, Italy)

On the other hand, papillomatous nevi show no structural change after accidental IPL treatment, except for a modest inflammation which generally tends to disappear within a few days. Shortly thereafter, dermal nevi look the same as before treatment.

In conclusion, the recognition of dermoscopic changes of the nevi after accidental exposure to luminous devices is important to exclude malignancy thus avoiding unnecessary excisions.

References

Álvarez-Garrido H, Garrido-Ríos AA, Martínez-Morán C, et al. Follow-up of melanocytic nevi after depilation techniques. J Cosmet Laser Ther. 2016;18:247–50.

Angermair J, Dettmar P, Linsenmann R, et al. Laser therapy of a dermal nevus in the esthetic zone of the nasal tip: a case report and comprehensive literature review. J Cosmet Laser Ther. 2015;17:296–300.

Argenziano G, Soyer HP, Chimenti S, et al. Dermoscopy of pigmented skin lesions: results of a consensus meeting via the Internet. J Am Acad Dermatol. 2003;48:679–93.

Arora H, Falto-Aizpurua L, Chacon A, et al. Lasers for nevi: a review. Lasers Med Sci. 2015;30:1991–2001.

Bray FN, Shah V, Nouri K. Laser treatment of congenital melanocytic nevi: a review of the literature. Lasers Med Sci. 2016;31:197–204.

Garrido-Ríos AA, Muñoz-Repeto I, Huerta-Brogeras M, et al. Dermoscopic changes in melanocytic nevi after depilation techniques. J Cosmet Laser Ther. 2013;15:98–101.

Hammes S, Raulin C, Karsai S, et al. Treating papillomatous intradermal nevi: lasers – yes or no? A prospective study. Hautarzt. 2008;59:101–7.

Köse O. Efficacy of the carbon dioxide fractional laser in the treatment of compound and dermal facial nevi using with dermatoscopic follow-up. J Dermatol Treat. 2018;19:1–5.

Martín JM, Monteagudo C, Bella R, et al. Complete regression of a melanocytic nevus under intense pulsed light therapy for axillary hair removal in a cosmetic center. Dermatology. 2012;224:193–7.

Ohmaru Y, Ohmaru K, Koga N, et al. New combined laser therapy for small mass of melanocytic nevi on the face. Laser Ther. 2011;20:301–6.

Omi T, Numano K. The role of the CO2 laser and fractional laser in Dermatology. Laser Ther. 2014;23:49–60.

Pampín Franco A, Gamo Villegas R, Floristán Muruzábal U, et al. Changes in melanocytic nevi after laser treatment evaluated by dermoscopy and reflectance confocal microscopy. Int J Dermatol. 2016;55:e307–9.

Sardana K. The science, reality, and ethics of treating common acquired melanocytic nevi (moles) with lasers. J Cutan Aesthet Surg. 2013;6:27.

Sillard L, Mantoux F, Larrouy JC, Hofman V, Passeron T, Lacour JP, et al. Dermoscopic changes of melanocytic nevi after laser hair removal. Eur J Dermatol. 2013;23:121–3.

Stratigos AJ, Dover JS, Arndt KA. Laser treatment of pigmented lesions--2000: how far have we gone? Arch Dermatol. 2000;136:915–21.

Zalaudek I, Argenziano G, Ferrara G, et al. Clinically equivocal melanocytic skin lesions with features of regression: a dermoscopic-pathological study. Br J Dermatol. 2004;150:64–71.

Zeng Y, Ji C, Zhan K, Weng W. Treatment of nasal ala nodular congenital melanocytic naevus with carbon dioxide laser and Q-switched Nd:YAG laser. Lasers Med Sci. 2016;31:1627–32.

Dermoscopy Applied to Lasers and IPL Treatments: Melasma, Seborrheic Keratoses, and Solar Lentigo

7

Melasma represents a common dermatological disorder of skin pigmentation that affects sun-exposed skin in females and which can also negatively influence the quality of life and cause substantial psychological and social distress. Whether this condition is acquired or genetic is still controversial; it clearly correlates with UV light exposure, a genetic predisposition, and hormonal variations (i.e., pregnancy, changes in uterine or ovarian hormones, oral contraceptives), but it can onset also in patients with hepatopathies and after cosmetic drug use (R. Yalamanchili et al. 2015).

For decades, the gold standard treatment for melasma has been represented by topical bleaching agents and strict photoprotection. Additional adjuvant treatment modalities include chemical peels and dermabrasion, all of which have demonstrated limited efficacy. Laser treatments gained good to excellent results depending on skin type and clinician's laser experience. Zoccali G. and collaborators (2010) tested Intense Pulsed Light devices on 38 patients with melasma: their results demonstrated that IPL stands out as an effective tool in the treatment and healing of a high percentage of hypermelanosis and melasma, with a very low risk of complications and an excellent satisfaction rate among patients (Fig. 7.1a–e).

Seborrheic keratoses (SK) represent one of the most common benign epidermal tumors observed by dermatologists in daily practice affecting at least 20% of the adult population, particularly the elderly (Roh et al. 2016). SK are often multiple, with great variability in terms of clinical presentation: size, clinical morphology, and color, even in the same individual with more SK (Yeatman et al. 1997).

They typically present as acquired, solitary, or multiple, well-demarcated brownish papules or plaques with a verrucous surface and predominantly occur on the head and neck area and on the trunk (Hafner and Vogt 2008). The diagnosis of SK is usually clinical; however, in certain cases differential diagnosis between SK and malignant melanoma is difficult. On dermoscopy, most of SK are characterized by the presence of comedo-like openings and milia-like cysts. Other criteria that

---

The contents of this book are partially based on the Italian language edition: "*The Usefulness of Dermoscopy in Laser and IPL Treatments*", Domenico Piccolo, © DEKA M.E.L.A Srl 2012.

© Springer Nature Switzerland AG 2020
D. Piccolo et al., *Quick Guide to Dermoscopy in Laser and IPL Treatments*,
https://doi.org/10.1007/978-3-319-41633-5_7

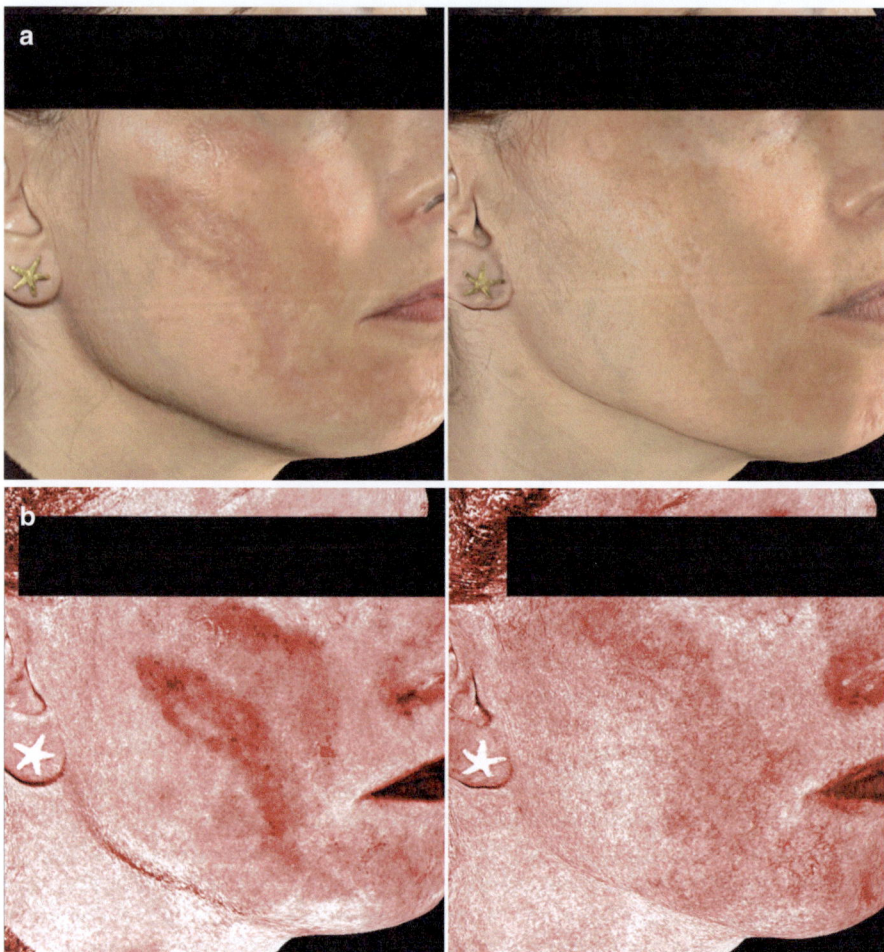

Fig. 7.1 (**a**) Melasma on the cheek on a facial scar of a young woman before any treatment and after 4QS laser sessions and one fractional treatment for the scar: excellent improvement is clinically observed. (**b**) The vascular software's filter highlights the consistent inflammatory response reductions after treatment. (**c**) The pigmentary software's filter highlights the consistent reduction of the melanin after treatment. (**d**) Comparison of frontal clinical images before any treatment (left) and after (right). (**e**) Comparison of frontal clinical images analyzed by the pigmentary filter before any treatment (left) and after (right). (Courtesy of Dr. Domenico Piccolo, Skin Center Avezzano, Italy)

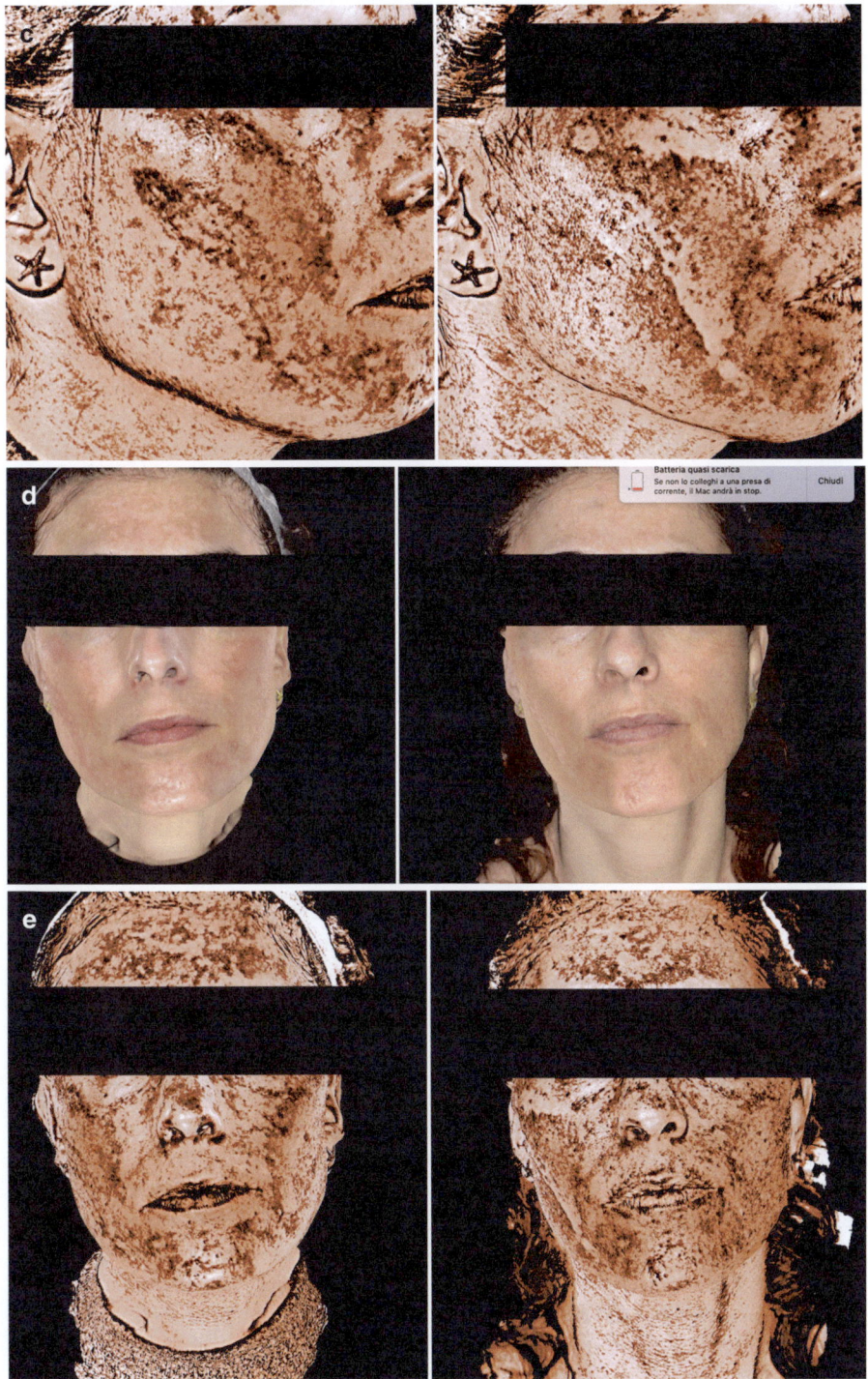

Fig. 7.1 (continued)

improve the diagnostic accuracy include hairpin blood vessels, fissures, sharp demarcation, and moth-eaten border (Kittler et al. 2016).

Although SK are biologically benign and do not require removal for medical reasons, many patients choose removal for aesthetic reasons (Del Rosso 2017). Current therapies for the treatment of SK are surgical or ablative removal. These include liquid nitrogen cryotherapy, shave removal, curettage, chemical peels, and certain laser modalities (Del Rosso 2017; Ranasinghe and Friedman 2017). Among the latter, it has been reported that ablative laser devices, such as the Er:YAG laser and the pulsed CO_2 laser, effectively treat SK through nonselective destruction of target tissues containing water (Fitzpatrick et al. 1994; Hafner and Vogt 2008; Krupashankar and IADVL Dermatosurgery Task Force 2008; Gurel and Aral 2015; Sayan et al. 2019).

Furthermore, nonablative lasers with selective photothermolysis, such as the QS 532-nm diode laser, the alexandrite laser QS 755-nm, and the Nd:YAG QS 532-/1064-nm lasers, have proven to be a valid therapeutic option for SK, theoretically aiming at the melanin pigments contained in SK as chromophores (Mehrabi and Brodell 2002; Kilmer 2002; Culbertson 2008; Kim et al. 2014).

In our opinion, the CO_2 represents the elective treatment for SK because its photo-coagulative action produces a precise wound with minimal blood loss, leaving a clean and dry surgical field. Dermoscopy performed before treatment detects the presence of classical SK patterns, such as comedo-like openings and milia-like cysts, the absence of a melanocytic pigment pattern, and, thus, the feasibility of treatment in the absence of a histological exam. The dermoscopic exam immediately after treatment demonstrates the disappearance of these patterns and the presence of small crusts and erythema. One month after the laser treatment, even though a clinical examination may diagnose the complete clearance of the lesion, the dermoscopic exam, especially in large-size SK, can highlight small residual areas of the lesion that can be successfully treated with a second session of laser therapy.

7.1   The Validity of Dermoscopy in the Treatment of Seborrheic Keratoses

In the case of small superficial and slightly pigmented seborrheic keratoses (up to 5 mm in diameter), IPL can be a valid therapeutic option since, thanks to its broad spectrum of action, it is possible to select the specific wavelength to act selectively on the pigment melanin of SK (Piccolo et al. 2014). Dermoscopy is useful either to confirm the diagnosis or to predict the outcome of the treatment. Immediately after the IPL, a color change from brown to gray is observed at dermoscopic evaluation, thus representing a sign of the success of the performed procedure. On the contrary, the absence of these changes testifies to its failure. When SK are successfully treated, they tend to disappear completely within 30 days after an average of two treatments. The dermoscopic analysis 30 days after the treatment is particularly difficult to perform since the result is the complete disappearance of the lesions without any residual erythema and therefore it is practically impossible to identify where the treated lesions were located. Lesions that do not respond to IPL treatment can therefore be treated with a CO_2 laser (Omi and Numano 2014).

7.2   The Validity of Dermoscopy in the Treatment of Solar Lentigines

Solar lentigines are benign hyperpigmented lesions that represent one of the first signs of photoaging. They generally appear during middle age and affect over 90% of Caucasians over the age of 60; however, 20% of Caucasians under the age of 35 have one or more solar lentils (Ortonne 1990). They derive from a variable degree of melanocyte proliferation and accumulation of melanin within keratinocytes in response to chronic exposure to UV radiations. Despite the benign lesions, solar lentigines are considered an independent risk factor for the development of melanoma (Bastiaens et al. 2004).

Solar lentigines are small, well-defined, round to oval, hyperpigmented lesions of sizes ranging from a few millimeters to more than a centimeter in diameter. They are mainly found on the face, the neck, the hands, and the forearms of adults and their number and size increase over time due to chronic exposure to the sun with a consequent increase in the transparency of the thinned and photodamaged skin.

The main concern in the treatment of solar lentigines is achieving the correct diagnosis. The diagnosis is usually based on the clinical characteristics; however, distinguishing a benign lentigo from other pigmented lesions can sometimes be challenging, even for experienced dermatologists. By identifying typical features of solar lentigines such as faint pigmented network, moth-eaten border, light brown fingerprint-like structures, or homogeneous pigmentation, dermoscopy greatly helps to rule out the correct diagnosis (Rosendahl et al. 2011; Zalaudek et al. 2013).

Solar lentigines are a significant cosmetic concern for many middle-aged and elderly patients with chronic accumulated sun exposure. Patients, particularly women, seeking for solar lentigines treatment account for a large part of dermatologic private practice. Available treatments consist of whitening agents (e.g., hydroquinone) (Dreher et al. 2011), retinoids (Draelos 2006; Kang et al. 2000), chemical peelings (e.g., trichloroacetic acid) as well as cryotherapy (Ortonne et al. 2006). Successful removal of these lesions can be also achieved with laser and non-laser light sources.

Up to now, laser treatment of solar lentigines is one of the most frequently performed cosmetic procedures in laser centers. According to the literature, among all pigmented lesions, solar lentigines show probably the best response to laser therapy. Generally, most of these lesions show more than 50% clinical lightening after one treatment session whereas complete eradication is usually observed after three treatments in 6- to 8-week intervals (Farris 2004; Stern et al. 1994; Bukvić Mokos et al. 2010). Recurrence is infrequent, but if the lesion is not completely clear, repigmentation is more likely (Kilmer and Garden 2000).

The short-pulsed QS lasers (QS alexandrite 750 nm, QS ruby 694 nm, and QS frequency-doubled Nd:YAG 532 nm) are the gold standard for the treatment of these lesions; however the long-pulsed counterparts could be an effective alternative, especially for patients with darker skin types (III–IV), since less cases of postinflammatory hyperpigmentation have occurred (Sebaratnam et al. 2014). Similarly, IPL devices have been successfully used for the treatment of solar freckles and at the same time they can improve diffuse photodamage and telangiectasias, making IPL a good treatment for general dyschromia regardless of its origin (Kawada et al. 2002; Ross et al. 2005; Piccolo et al. 2014).

In our routine clinical practice, IPL is used for the treatment of solar lentigines associated with photoaging (Figs. 7.2a, 7.3a, 7.4a, 7.5a, and 7.6). The dermoscopic exam performed before IPL treatment shows the typical aspect of solar lentigo such as the pseudo-network and moth-eaten border (Figs. 7.2b, 7.3b, 7.4b, 7.5b, and 7.6). The dermoscopic sign indicating therapeutic success immediately after one treatment with IPL is the color change from brown to gray (Fig. 7.4c). The pigmentary software's filter analysis can also highlight the therapeutic success by comparing the first clinical image (Fig. 7.2c) with the clinical presentation at the time of the last follow-up visit (Fig. 7.2d). In the case of solar lentigo on the back due to photodamage, the dermoscopic examination performed immediately after IPL treatment shows an increase in pigmentation associated with a white halo all around the clinically prominent edges of the lesion. These phenomena are indications of therapeutic success. The presence of the peripheral white halo is a characteristic feature of solar lentigo of the trunk while it cannot be observed in those on the hands or face.

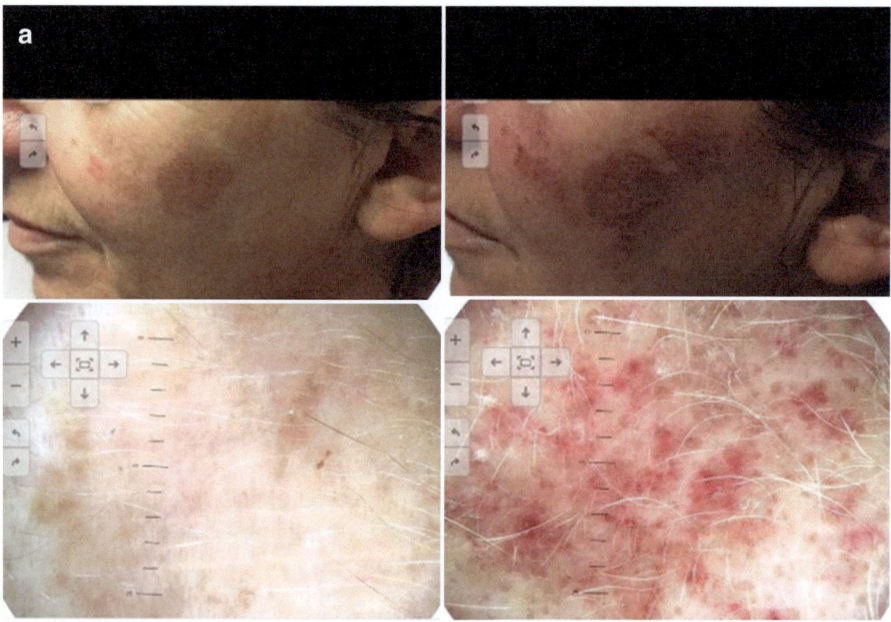

Fig. 7.2 (**a**) Clinical and dermoscopical images of a solar lentigo on the cheek of a woman before (up on the left and down on the left) and after 1QS session (up on the right and down on the right). (**b**) Clinical and dermoscopical images of a solar lentigo on the cheek of a woman before (up on the left and down on the left) and after 3 months after the treatment (up on the right and down on the right). (**c**) Comparison of clinical images before any treatment (left) and after (right): an excellent aesthetic outcome has been achieved. (**d**) Comparison of clinical images analyzed by the pigmentary filter before any treatment (left) and after (right): a consistent reduction of the melanin is observed. (Courtesy of Dr. Domenico Piccolo, Skin Center Avezzano, Italy)

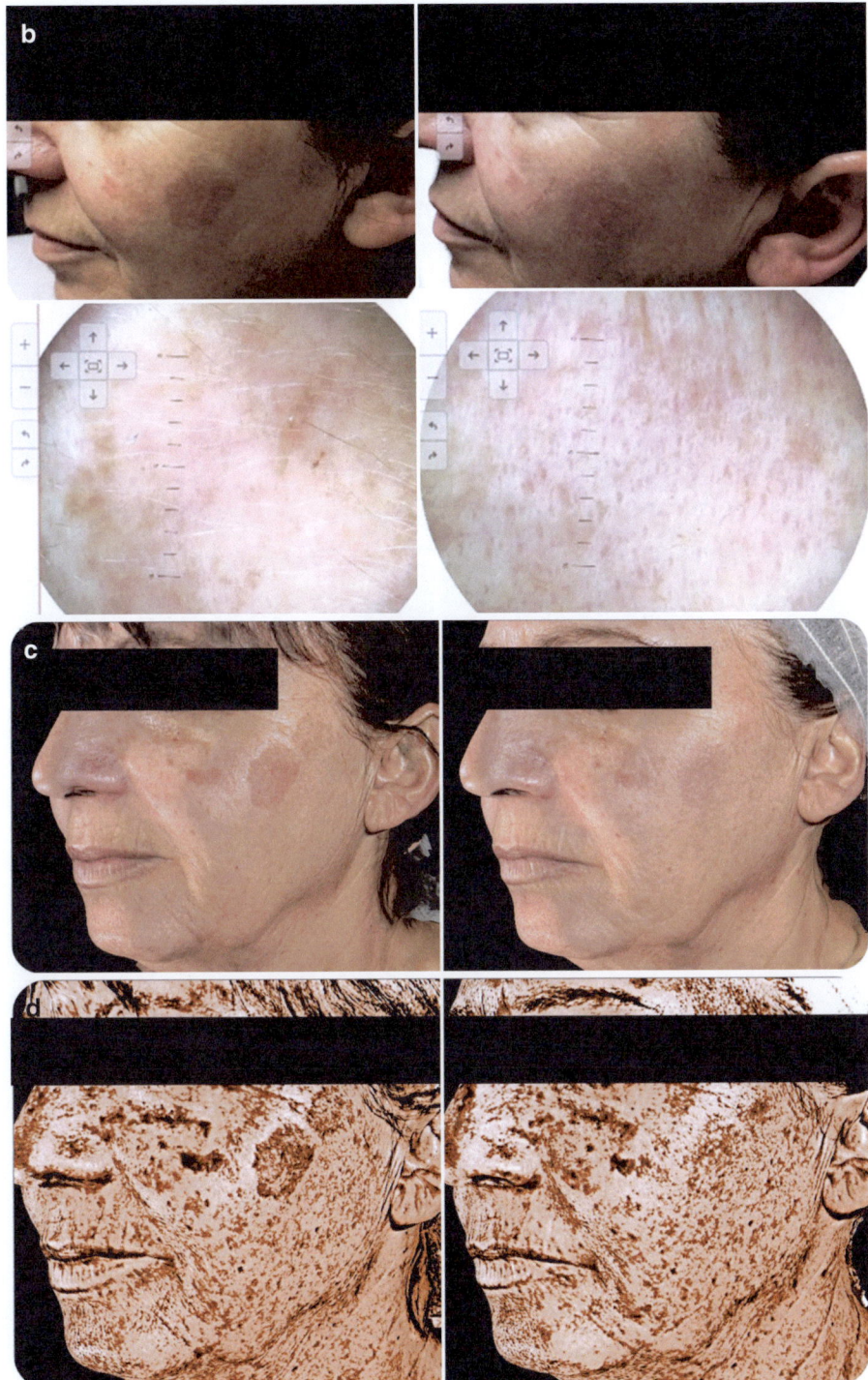

Fig. 7.2 (continued)

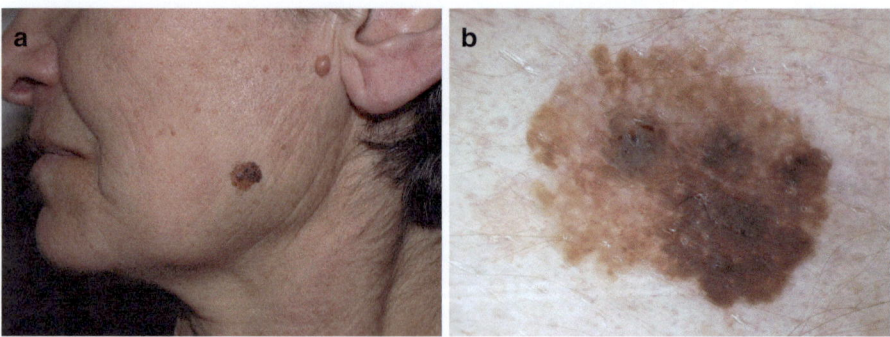

Fig. 7.3 (**a**) Clinical presentation of a solar lentigo in an old woman. (**b**) Dermoscopic exam helps the clinician to confirm the diagnosis. (Courtesy of Dr. Domenico Piccolo, Skin Center Avezzano, Italy)

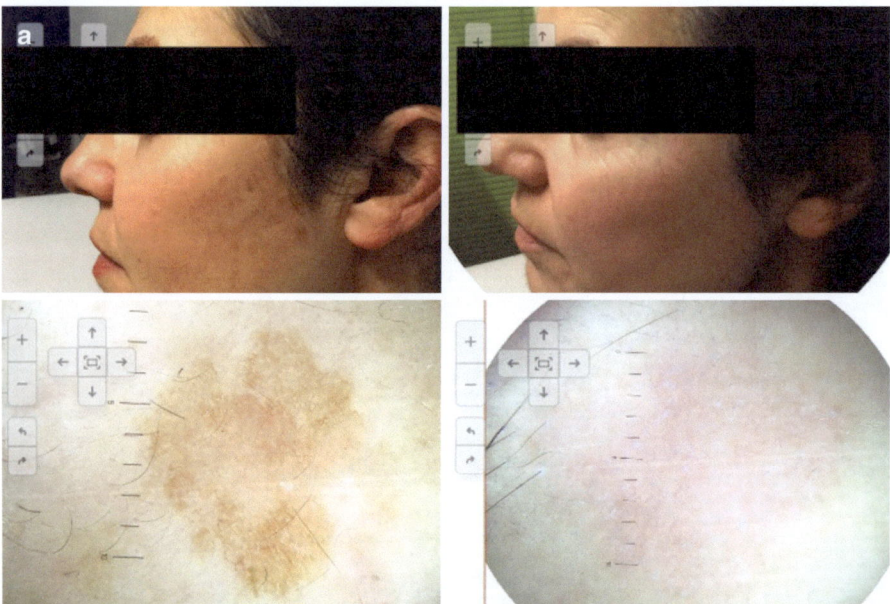

Fig. 7.4 (**a, b**) Clinical presentation of a solar lentigo presented on the face of a young woman. Dermoscopic exam performed before and after treatment highlights the clearance of the lesion. (**c**) Clinical presentation of the lesion and dermoscopic exam performed before and immediately after 1QS session. (Courtesy of Dr. Domenico Piccolo, Skin Center Avezzano, Italy)

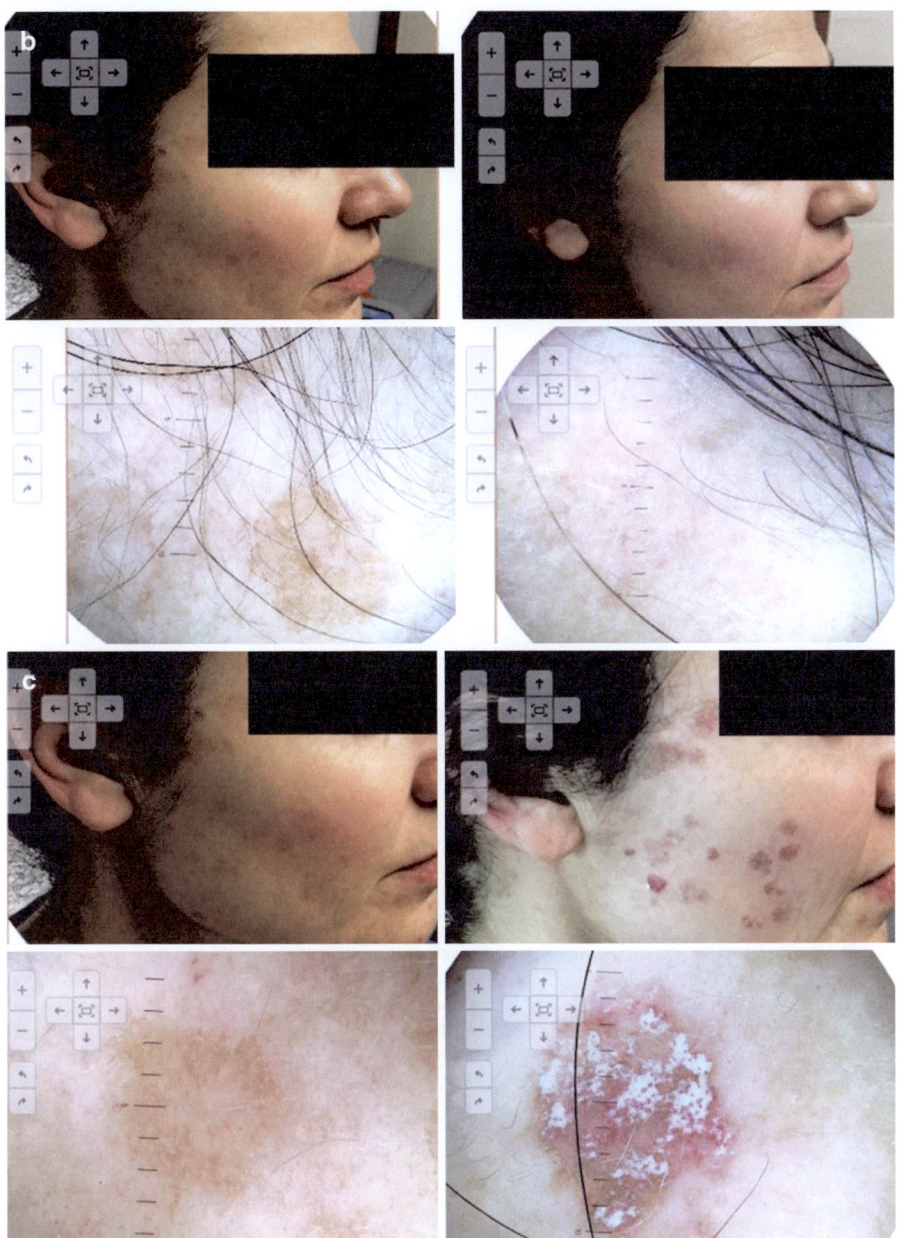

Fig. 7.4 (continued)

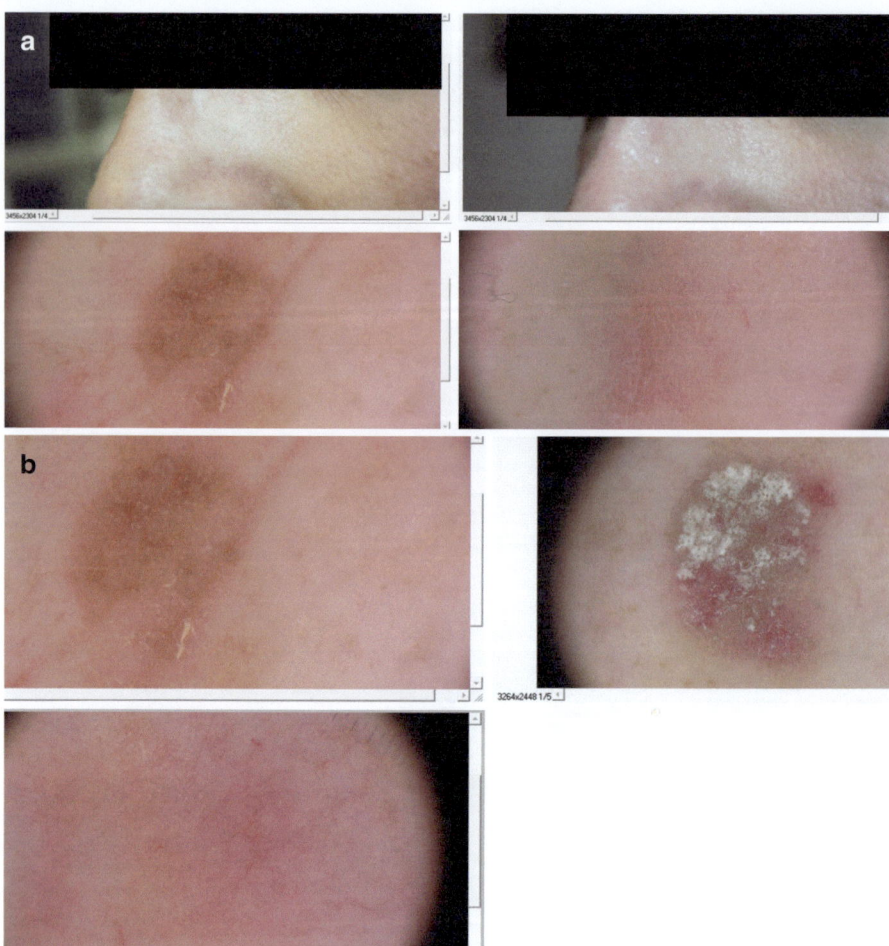

Fig. 7.5 (**a**) Solar lentigo on the nose of a young woman. The dermoscopic exam performed before IPL treatment shows the typical aspect of solar lentigo such as the pseudo-network and moth-eaten border. (**b**) The dermoscopic sign indicating therapeutic success immediately after one treatment with IPL is the color change from brown to gray. (Courtesy of Dr. Domenico Piccolo, Skin Center Avezzano, Italy)

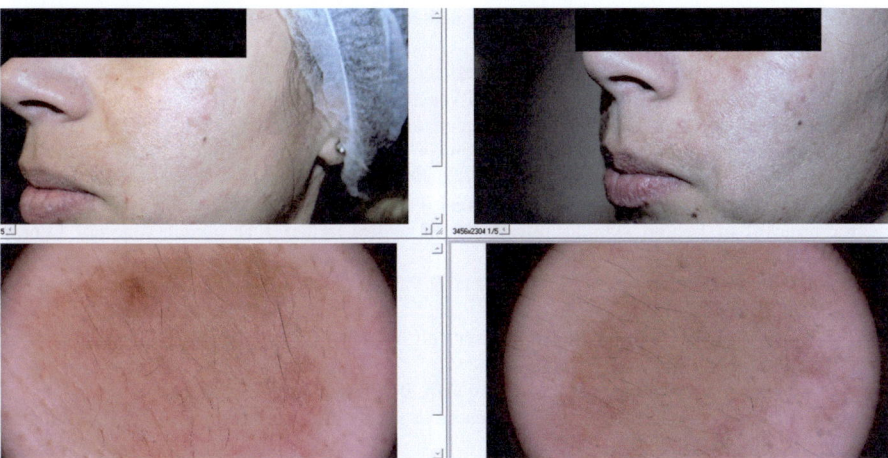

Fig. 7.6 Solar lentigo on the cheek of a young woman before and after a QS treatment. The dermoscopic exam before the treatment confirm the diagnosis; the dermoscopic exam performed after the first IPL treatment confirmed the improvement of the lesion and suggests performing another session to achieve the complete clearance of the lentigo. (Courtesy of Dr. Domenico Piccolo, Skin Center Avezzano, Italy)

References

Bastiaens M, Hoefnagel J, Westendorp R, et al. Solar lentigines are strongly related to sun exposure in contrast to ephelides. Pigment Cell Res. 2004;17:225–9.

Bukvić Mokos Z, Lipozenčić J, Ceović R, et al. Laser therapy of pigmented lesions: pro and contra. Acta Dermatovenerol Croat. 2010;18:185–9.

Culbertson GR. 532-nm diode laser treatment of seborrheic keratoses with color enhancement. Dermatol Surg. 2008;34:525–8.

Del Rosso JQ. A Closer look at seborrheic keratoses: patient perspectives, clinical relevance, medical necessity, and implications for management. J Clin Aesthet Dermatol. 2017;10:16–25.

Draelos ZD. The combination of 2% 4-hydroxyanisole (mequinol) and 0.01% tretinoin effectively improves the appearance of solar lentigines in ethnic groups. J Cosmet Dermatol. 2006;5:239–44.

Dreher F, Draelos ZD, Gold MH, et al. Efficacy of hydroquinone-free skin-lightening cream for photoaging. J Cosmet Dermatol. 2011;12:12–7.

Farris PK. Combination therapy for solar lentigines. J Drugs Dermatol. 2004;3:S23–6.

Fitzpatrick RE, Goldman MP, Ruiz-Esparza J. Clinical advantage of the CO2 laser superpulsed mode. Treatment of verruca vulgaris, seborrheic keratoses, lentigines, and actinic cheilitis. J Dermatol Surg Oncol. 1994;20:449–56.

Gurel MS, Aral BB. Effectiveness of erbium:YAG laser and cryosurgery in seborrheic keratoses: randomized, prospective intraindividual comparison study. J Dermatol Treat. 2015;26:477–80.

Hafner C, Vogt T. Seborrheic keratosis. [Article in English, German]. J Deutschen Dermatologischen Gesellschaft. 2008;6:664–77.

Kang S, Goldfarb MT, Weiss JS, et al. Assessment of adapalene gel for the treatment of actinic keratoses and lentigines: a randomized trial. J Am Acad Dermatol. 2000;49:83–90.

Kawada A, Shiraishi H, Asai M, et al. Clinical improvement of solar lentigines and ephelides with an intense pulsed light source. Dermatol Surg. 2002;28:504–8.

Kilmer SL. Laser eradication of pigmented lesions and tattoos. Dermatol Clin. 2002;20:37–53.

Kilmer SL, Garden JM. Laser treatment of pigmented lesions and tattoos. Semin Cutan Med Surg. 2000;19(4):232–44.

Kim YK, Kim DY, Lee SJ, et al. Therapeutic efficacy of long-pulsed 755-nm alexandrite laser for seborrheic keratoses. J Eur Acad Dermatol Venereol. 2014;28:1007–11.

Kittler H, Marghoob AA, Argenziano G, et al. Standardization of terminology in dermoscopy/ dermatoscopy: results of the third consensus conference of the International Society of Dermoscopy. J Am Acad Dermatol. 2016;74:1093–11.

Krupashankar DS, IADVL Dermatosurgery Task Force. Standard guidelines of care: CO2 laser for removal of benign skin lesions and resurfacing. Indian J Dermatol Venereol Leprol. 2008;74(Suppl):S61–7.

Mehrabi D, Brodell RT. Use of the alexandrite laser for treatment of seborrheic keratoses. Dermatol Surg. 2002;28:437–9.

Omi T, Numano K. The role of the CO2 laser and fractional laser in Dermatology. Laser Ther. 2014;23:49–60.

Ortonne JP. Pigmentary changes of the ageing skin. Br J Dermatol. 1990;122:21–8.

Ortonne JP, Pandya AG, Lui H, et al. Treatment of solar lentigines. J Am Acad Dermatol. 2006;54(suppl 2):S262–71.

Piccolo D, Di Marcantonio D, Crisman G, et al. Unconventional use of intense pulsed light. Biomed Res Int. 2014;2014:618206.

Ranasinghe GC, Friedman AJ. Managing seborrheic keratoses: evolving strategies for optimizing patient outcomes. J Drugs Dermatol. 2017;16:1064–8.

Roh NK, Hahn HJ, Lee YW, et al. Clinical and histopathological investigation of seborrheic keratosis. Ann Dermatol. 2016;28:152–8.

Rosendahl C, Tschandl P, Cameron A, et al. Diagnostic accuracy of dermatoscopy for melanocytic and nonmelanocytic pigmented lesions. J Am Acad Dermatol. 2011;64:1068–73.

Ross EV, Smirnov M, Pankratov M, Altshuler G. Intense pulsed light and laser treatment of facial telangiectasias and dyspigmentation: some theoretical and practical comparisons. Dermatol Surg. 2005;31(9 Pt 2):1188–98.

Sayan A, Sindel A, Ethunandan M, et al. Management of seborrhoeic keratosis and actinic keratosis with an erbium:YAG laser-experience with 547 patients. Int J Oral Maxillofac Surg. 2019;48:902. pii: S0901-502730341-2.

Sebaratnam DF, Lim AC, Lowe PM, et al. Lasers and laser-like devices: part two. Aust J Dermatol. 2014;55:1–14.

Stern RS, Dover JS, Levin JA, et al. Laser therapy versus cryotherapy of lentigines: a comparative trial. J Am Acad Dermatol. 1994;30:985–7.

Yalamanchili R, Shastry V, Betkerur J. Clinicoepidemiological study and quality of life assessment in melasma. Indian J Dermatol. 2015;60(5):519.

Yeatman JM, Kilkenny M, Marks R. The prevalence of seborrheic keratoses in an Australian population: does exposure to sunlight play a part in their frequency? Br J Dermatol. 1997;137:411–4.

Zalaudek I, Lallas A, Longo C, et al. Problematic lesions in the elderly. Dermatol Clin. 2013;31:549–64.

Zoccali G, Piccolo D, Allegra P, et al. Melasma treated with intense pulsed light. Aesthet Plast Surg. 2010;34(4):486–93.

8

Dermoscopy Applied to Laser and IPL Treatments: Telangiectasias

Telangiectasias are defined as broken or widened small blood vessels sited underneath the surface of the skin (or mucous membrane) creating a visible pattern of red-violet lines, virtually anywhere on the body, often occurring in fair-skinned patients with long-term sun damage.

Generally, they represent mainly an aesthetic problem but they could also be the sign of a more severe medical condition, due to several causes (connective tissue diseases, vascular diseases, etc.), thus warranting a closer inspection. Even though the etiology remains mainly unknown, some predisposing factors have been identified:

- Genetics
- Prolonged use of topical or oral corticosteroids
- Hormonal changes (pregnancy, menopause, oral contraceptives)
- Long history of sun and wind exposure
- Excessive alcohol consumption
- Direct skin trauma (including surgical incisions)
- Skin diseases (acne, psoriasis)
- Venous insufficiency (varicose veins)

Some severe medical conditions could be implied as well in the occurring of telangiectasias, such as:

- Liver diseases (cirrhosis)
- Xeroderma pigmentosum (XP)
- Osler–Weber–Rendu disease
- Ataxia telangiectasia (AT)
- Sturge–Weber syndrome

The contents of this book are partially based on the Italian language edition: "*The Usefulness of Dermoscopy in Laser and IPL Treatments*", Domenico Piccolo, © DEKA M.E.L.A Srl 2012.

© Springer Nature Switzerland AG 2020
D. Piccolo et al., *Quick Guide to Dermoscopy in Laser and IPL Treatments*,
https://doi.org/10.1007/978-3-319-41633-5_8

- Vascular malformation (port-wine stains (PWS), spider angiomas)
- Klippel–Trenaunay–Weber (KTW)
- Bloom syndrome
- Scleroderma
- Lupus erythematosus
- Dermatomyositis

So many medical conditions can lead to telangiectasias, and new laser technologies are available to treat these conditions.

8.1   Treatment Options

Intense pulsed light, especially in its Rhodamine variant (Piccolo et al. 2016), and Nd:YAG are the gold standard treatment. Usually, a complete treatment protocol can require one to four IPL or laser sessions, depending on the needs (Myers et al. 2005; Ciocon et al. 2009; Babilas et al. 2010).

Nd:YAG laser is without doubt an excellent instrument for treating facial telangiectasias. In particular, the increased penetration depth is extremely useful for treating vessels located on the face where treatment with IPL is less effective, such as on the wings of the nose. The results are quite similar to those of IPL. Like most other light sources, there is the risk of scarring or dichromic effects by the use of inappropriate fluence or pulse lengths (Erceg et al. 2013; Salem et al. 2013; Shim and Abdullah 2013).

The current dye lasers, which use rhodamine as the active medium, allow producing wavelengths ranging between 585 and 600 nm. These wavelengths allow obtaining deeper penetration into the tissues to treat even lesions morphologically distributed in depth, while maintaining high hemoglobin selectivity. The undisputed therapeutic advantage of these wavelengths, linked to the hemoglobin absorption selectivity, which makes dye laser the gold standard in vascular lesion treatment, can however create some discomfort in the treatment of aesthetic disorders because of the possible formation of purple bruises.

In addition, technological innovation has introduced pulsed light systems, which allow for broadband emissions, with a spectrum of wavelengths ranging between 500 and 1200 nm. The advantage of pulsed light systems lies in the fact that they allow hitting the target of the vascular component over several wavelengths, exploiting both the components of the above mentioned laser systems and other wavelengths that fall within their emission spectrum. The largest limit of pulsed light in vascular treatment is linked to its constructive technology, which leads to higher energy emission in the infrared, leaving a lower percentage of light energy in the visible emission, where both the hemoglobin absorption peaks and typical wavelengths of dye laser systems are located. Moreover, the emission over the entire visible spectrum involves the pigmentary component in the skin tissue, which covers the entire visible spectrum with greater selectivity for increasingly shorter wavelengths. The Right Light technology handpiece, on the SynchroVasQ platform, is a pulsed light system that allows enhancing emission performance in the wavelength range between 550 and 650 nm, in order to obtain pulsed light performance closer to dye lasers, thereby creating an effective and more comfortable treatment. The system uses rhodamine as a fluorescent substance that can absorb the wavelengths in the UV spectrum up to 550 nm and emit them again in fluorescence within a range between 550 and 650 nm, with a rhodamine peak around 570 nm, without losing energy during this transformation. All this allows obtaining an amount of energy that falls within the range between 550 and 650 nm greater than traditional pulsed light systems, which translates into higher performance on vascular lesions.

Seven years ago we started to test another source of IPL; a new pulsed light optimized for the 595 nm dye wavelength has been used thanks to the RightLight Technology (SynchroVasQ, DekaMela, Italy). This new kind of IPL, the so-called Rhodamine IPL (r-IPL), has wavelengths optimized for 595 nm, a maximum fluence of 25 J/cm^2, and pulse duration ranging from 3 to 24 ms. Two different spot sizes of 2 and 6 cm^2 are available. Epidermal cooling is provided by the handpiece (Piccolo 2012; Piccolo et al. 2016).

We treated 20 patients (15 females and five males) aged between 38 and 68 years (average age 52.3 years) with Fitzpatrick phototype II–III for the telangiectatic component of acne rosacea (Fig. 8.1a, b).

We chose the 500 nm handpiece; fluence, 12–16 J/cm^2; double pulse mode, 5–10 ms in duration; interpulse delay, 10 ms with epidermal cooling already provided by the IPL handpiece. The papulo-pustular component was subsequently treated with the 550 nm handpiece; fluence, 10–12 J/cm^2; double pulse mode, 5–10 ms in duration; interpulse delay, 10 ms with epidermal cooling already provided by the IPL handpiece.

Patients required from two up to five sessions, at intervals of approximately 20–30 days, to gain significant results, even though a moderate reduction in vessel number and size and a partial disappearance of papules was observed subsequent to the second session. During the 5-year follow-up, we gained a complete absence of recurrences and the persistence of the achieved outcomes in 17/20 patients (85%) whereas the other three patients required a new treatment within the year for the slight relapse of the papulo-pustular component.

We then treated 45 patients affected by facial telangiectasias with r-IPL set as follows: fluence range between 18 and 23 J/cm^2, double pulse at 8 ms, and a delay of 10 ms between pulses. Two sessions required. Any epidermal cooling during the treatment, apart from that incorporated in the handpieces, has been administered since patients' burning sensation was referred from mild to moderate. In our experience, all patients reported the absence of side effects, such as intense erythema and slight crusting noticed with the r-IPL device at conservative parameters (first pass), thus leading to increase the fluence (second pass) to achieve marked results with reduced number of sessions.

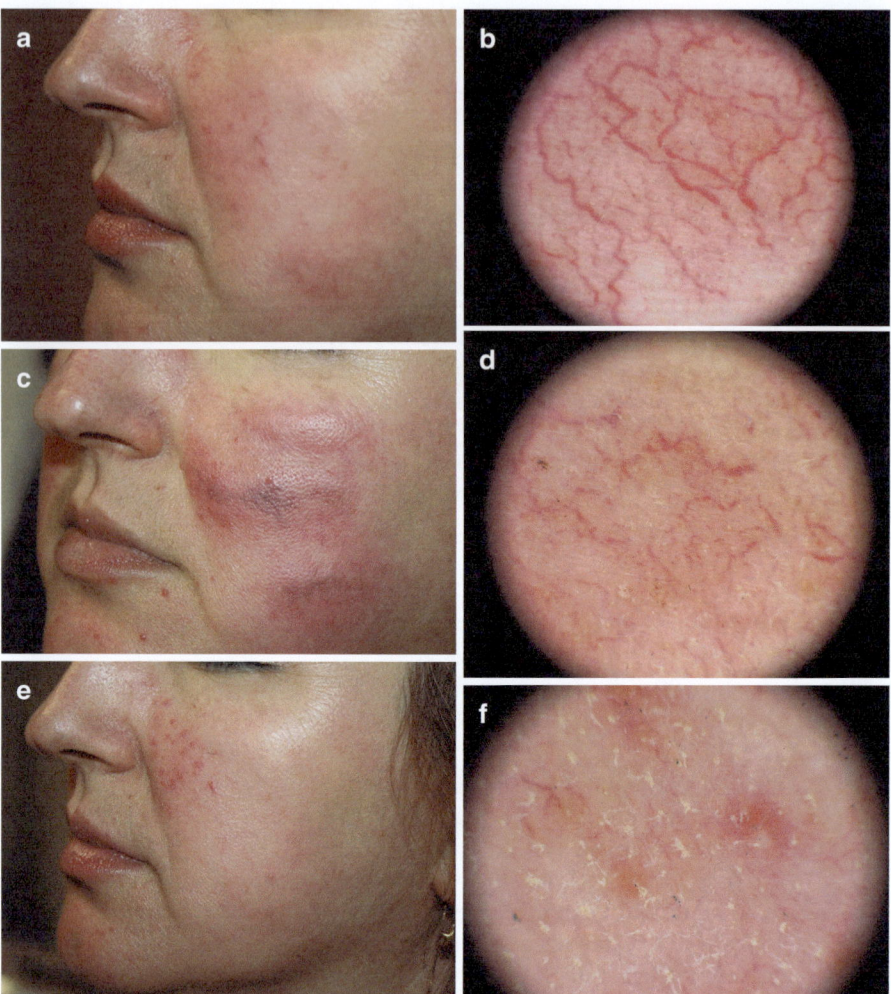

Fig. 8.1 (**a**) Clinical picture of telangiectasias in acne rosacea of a young man before any treatment. (**b**) Dermoscopy performed before any treatment is useful to highlight the number and gauge of the ectatic vessels. (**c**) Clinical image taken immediately after treatment. (**d**) The dermoscopic exam performed immediately after treatment reveals the color change from red to blue. In the areas where vessels persist, more than one session may be necessary as it is possible that vessels which resisted in the first treatment will disappear in the following session. (**e**) Clinical image after four IPL sessions. (**f**) The excellent clinical results are confirmed using dermoscopy with the complete clearance of the ecstatic vessels. (Courtesy of Dr. Domenico Piccolo, Skin Center Avezzano, Italy)

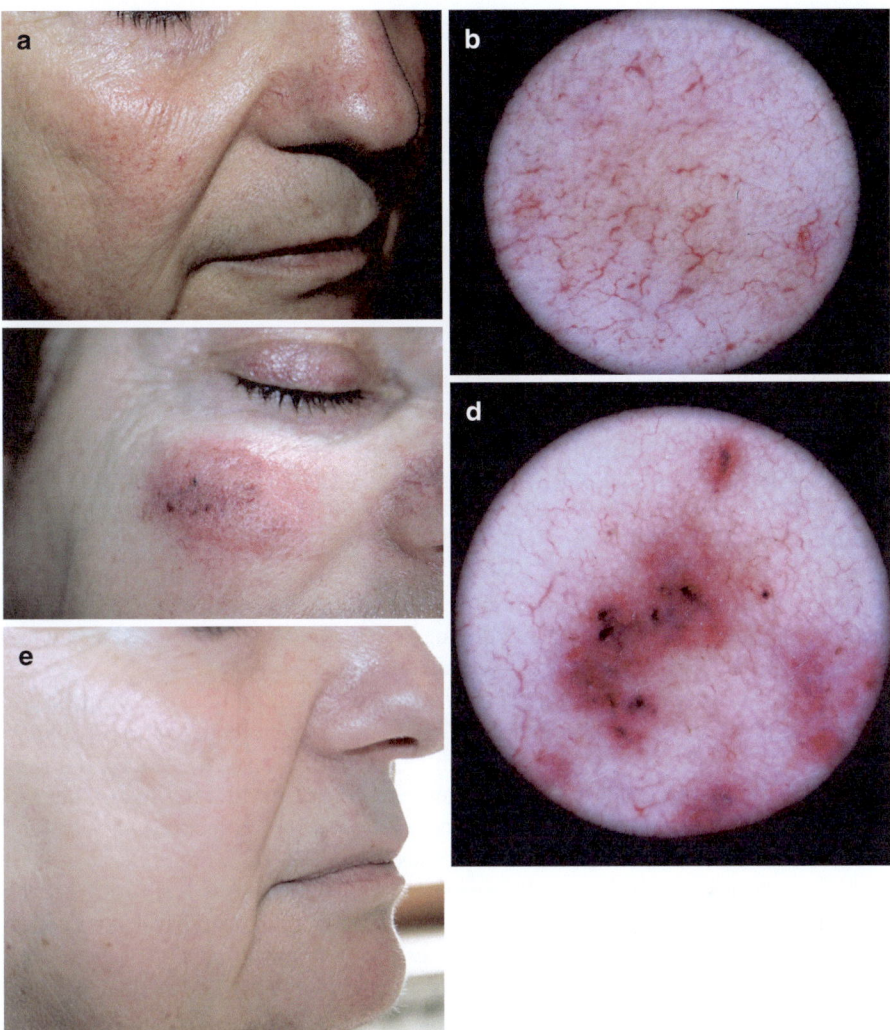

Fig. 8.2 (**a**) Clinical picture of telangiectasis in acne rosacea of a middle-age woman before any treatment. (**b**) Dermoscopy performed before any treatment is useful to highlight the number and gauge of the ectatic vessels. (**c**) Clinical image taken immediately after a first IPL treatment. (**d**) The dermoscopic exam performed immediately after the first IPL treatment reveals damage to the vessels. (**e**) Clinical image after three IPL sessions with an excellent clinical result. (Courtesy of Dr. Domenico Piccolo, Skin Center Avezzano, Italy)

8.2   The Validity of Dermoscopy in the Treatment of Telangiectasias

The dermoscopy exam performed immediately after a laser or IPL treatment states the reduction in number of the vessels in case of partial resolution, thus meaning that another session is suggested (Fig. 8.1c, d), and a disappearance of all telangiectatic structures in case of complete healing (Fig. 8.1e, f).

In case of telangiectasias sited on the lower limb, dermoscopy is essentially the choice of the gauge and the number of vessels which are usually not clearly visible to the naked eye.

Dermoscopy performed immediately after treatment shows the contraction of the vessels with total or partial disappearance of the treated vessels. Few days after, dermoscopy highlights some vessels' damage in the form of small scabs, thus resulting from the necrosis of the vessels' walls. The presence of small scabs along the length of the vessel is predictive of a good clinical result, which will be clearly visible 30–45 days after treatment. Meanwhile, it is important not to perform another session before this interval period in the aim to achieve a complete healing (Sevila et al. 2004; Piccolo et al. 2016).

On dermoscopy, telangiectasia highlights enlarged and broken superficial blood vessels and quantifies the number and gauge of the vessels to be treated as well as the concomitant presence of any photodamage (Fig. 8.2a, b).

Excellent results have been gained by using IPL and, particularly, Rhodamine IPL in facial and nasal telangiectasias. Vessels treated can react to the IPL with a coagulation or with a contraction. In both cases, dermoscopy performed immediately after each session could show a change in color from red to blue (in case of coagulation) or the complete disappearance of the vessel (contraction), thus leading to a good prediction of the aesthetic outcomes (Piccolo 2012) (Fig. 8.2c, d).

Using dermoscopy before each laser session is important as well: in a 2-week interval period from one session to another, a dermoscopy exam performed before each treatment demonstrates the gradual decrease in number and size of the treated vessels. These dermoscopic modifications correspond in a high percentage of cases to excellent clinical results (Piccolo et al. 2014) (Fig. 8.2e).

References

Babilas P, Schreml S, Szeimies RM, et al. Intense pulsed light (IPL): a review. Lasers Surg Med. 2010;42(2):93–104.

Ciocon DH, Boker A, Goldberg DJ. Intense pulsed light: what works, what's new, what's next. Facial Plast Surg. 2009;25(5):290–300.

Erceg A, de Jong EM, van de Kerkhof PC, et al. The efficacy of pulsed dye laser treatment for inflammatory skin diseases: a systematic review. J Am Acad Dermatol. 2013;69(4):609–615.e8.

Myers P, Bowler P, Hills S. A retrospective study of the efficacy of intense pulsed light for the treatment of dermatologic disorders presenting to a cosmetic skin clinic. J Cosmet Dermatol. 2005;4(4):262–6.

Piccolo D. The usefulness of dermoscopy in laser and intense pulsed light treatments. Florence: Remo Sandron Edition; 2012.

Piccolo D, Crisman G, Kostaki D, et al. Rhodamine intense pulsed light versus conventional pulsed light for facial teleangiectasias. J Cosmet Laser Ther. 2016;18(2):80–5.

Piccolo D, Di Marcantonio D, Crisman G, et al. Unconventional use of intense pulsed light. Biomed Res Int. 2014;2014:618206.

Salem SA, Abdel Fattah NS, Tantawy SM, et al. Neodymium-yttrium aluminum garnet laser versus pulsed dye laser in erythemato-telangiectatic rosacea: comparison of clinical efficacy and effect on cutaneous substance (P) expression. J Cosmet Dermatol. 2013;12(3):187–94.

Sevila A, Nagore E, Botella-Estrada R, et al. Videomicroscopy of venular malformations (port-wine stain type): prediction of response to pulsed dye laser. Pediatr Dermatol. 2004;21(5):589–96.

Shim TN, Abdullah A. The effect of pulsed dye laser on the dermatology life quality index in erythematotelangiectatic rosacea patients: an assessment. J Clin Aesthet Dermatol. 2013;6(4):30–2.

Dermoscopy Applied to Laser and IPL Treatments: Flat Angiomas and Port-Wine Stains

9

Port-wine stains (PWSs), also known as nevus flammeus, are the most common congenital vascular malformations, with an incidence of 0.3–0.5% of all newborns worldwide (Jacobs and Walton 1976). They account for 1.4% of all vascular lesions seen in newborns (Osburn et al. 1987). PWSs are usually isolated skin abnormalities, but in rare cases, they may be part of complex malformation syndromes such as Sturge–Weber syndrome or Klippel–Trénaunay–Weber syndrome.

PWSs usually begin as unilateral cutaneous or mucosal lesions with irregular borders and inhomogeneous colors ranging from pink to red to violet. Over 40% of PWSs are located on the face following the trigeminal nerve (fifth cranial nerve) distribution (branches 1–3 or V1–3) (Enjolras et al. 1985), but they can affect any part of the body, particularly the neck, upper trunk, arms, and legs. PWSs are characterized by an increase in the number of ectatic capillaries, affecting either the dermal papillae capillary loops, the horizontal plexus at the dermal–subcutaneous junction, or a combination, which result in increased hemoglobin content in the overlying skin. The depth and size of these vessels significantly reflect the clinical appearance of PWSs: brighter red lesions are usually composed of dilated superficial vessels, faint pink lesions are composed by small deep vessels, and purple lesions are composed by large deep vessels (Haliasos et al. 2013).

PWSs do not involute over time but may gradually progress and evolve into lifelong lesions. PWS lesions do not proliferate and grow, but if untreated, they may demonstrate chronic vascular dilatation becoming darker, raised, and nodular (Finley et al. 1984). Hypertrophy is a common development in PWSs affecting nearly two-thirds of patients by the fifth decade of life (Geronemus and Ashinoff 1991). Its prevalence increases with age, and the peak age of onset has been reported between 20 and 39 years (Klapman and Yao 2001; van Drooge et al. 2012). While the size and distribution of the lesions do not change with age, increased age correlates with progressive vascular ectasia and color shifts from pink to purple (Barsky et al. 1980).

The contents of this book are partially based on the Italian language edition: *"The Usefulness of Dermoscopy in Laser and IPL Treatments"*, Domenico Piccolo, © DEKA M.E.L.A Srl 2012.

© Springer Nature Switzerland AG 2020
D. Piccolo et al., *Quick Guide to Dermoscopy in Laser and IPL Treatments*,
https://doi.org/10.1007/978-3-319-41633-5_9

Hypertrophy may be either diffuse thickened, namely cobblestone pattern, or nodular (Klapman and Yao 2001; van Drooge et al. 2012). The cobblestoning appearance of PWSs may be a result of localized pronounced vascular ectasia and proliferations of thin- and/or thick-walled vessels and their stroma as well as numerous epithelial, neural, and mesenchymal hamartomatous abnormalities (Finley et al. 1984).

Both diffuse thickened and nodular PWSs have been associated with increased risk of spontaneous bleeding, loss of function, and increasing disfigurement. Regarding PWS involving the first branch of trigeminal nerve, the most frequent ocular comorbidity is glaucoma with a prevalence rate ranging from 30% to 70% (Wu et al. 2017). In addition, PWSs can be rarely associated with basal cell carcinoma (Silapunt et al. 2004), pyogenic granulomas (Sheehan et al. 2004), and squamous cell carcinoma (Rajan et al. 2006).

While PWSs are usually considered congenital vascular lesions, a few cases of acquired PWSs have also been described in the literature (Bansal et al. 2015; Freysz et al. 2013; Adams and Lucky 2000; Colver and Ryan 1986). Acquired WPSs are clinically and pathologically similar to their congenital counterparts (Salim et al. 2003). Most of them are idiopathic or secondary to a mechanical trauma (Senti and Trüeb 2000). Other underlying causes include actinic exposure, pregnancy, drugs, tumors, frostbite injury, cluster headache, acoustic neuroma, and obstruction of a peritoneovenous shunt and herpes zoster infection (Bansal et al. 2015; Hoque and Holden 2005; Adams and Lucky 2000; Colver and Ryan 1986).

Whether congenital or acquired PWSs the exact pathogenetic mechanism has yet to be elucidated. The most accepted hypothesis is a maturational defect of local sympathetic nerves resulting in a loss of normal vascular tone which lead to continue blood flow and therefore to vascular ectasia typically seen in PWSs (Rosen and Smoller 1987; Lanigan and Cotterill 1990). Mutations in RASA1 and vascular endothelial growth factor (VEGF) have been also implicated in the pathogenesis and progression of PWSs (Hershkovitz et al. 2008; Vural et al. 2008). Regarding trauma-related PWSs, it has been proposed that injury may affect a previously effective local vascular innervation leading to the development of these lesions (Adams and Lucky 2000).

Although most PWS lesions are not life-threatening, lifelong persistence and progressive worsening with the patient's age can lead to aesthetic and functional compromises. The visible manifestation of PWSs is often considered a disfigurement and the accompanying social stigma often causes emotional and psychological distress in affected individuals and their families (Malm and Carlberg 1988; Lanigan and Cotterill 1989). Patients with PWSs have a profound sense of embarrassment and shame, as well as low levels of self-esteem, reflecting on development of social skills. Several studies have reported that the presence of PWSs has a significant negative impact on quality of life (QoL) (van der Horst et al. 1997; Masnari et al. 2013; Hagen et al. 2017), thus suggesting that this disorder is not merely an aesthetic skin problem. The burden of having a PWS is equivalent of other dermatologic conditions. Hagen and collaborators (2017) measured QoL in 244 patients with facial PWS using a Skindex-29 instrument and found that the composite dermatologic-specific QoL scores were similar to those of cutaneous T-cell lymphoma, rosacea, alopecia, and vitiligo. In this study, younger patients had a greater impairment of quality of life, particularly with respect to emotions, compared to their older counterparts.

9.1   Treatment Options

Nowadays, PWS management remains a challenge. The rationale for treatment of patients with PWSs is based on the concept that early laser intervention may reduce the likelihood and severity of unwanted associated effects such as hypertrophy, spontaneous bleeding, disfigurement as well as psychosocial morbidity (Hagen et al. 2017). Although current treatment protocols, such as vascular-selective lasers, have been shown to be effective in the treatment of PWSs, these treatments are far from being optimal. According to the literature, 12–85% of PWS patients achieve less than 50% clearance, of the lesions, regardless of the treatment modality (Chen et al. 2012; Astner and Anderson 2005).

Pulsed dye laser, Nd:YAG, alexandrite, and the diode laser are the most used lasers in the treatment of PWSs (Li et al. 2010; Burns and Navarro 2009). Among them, pulsed dye laser (PDL, 595 nm) represents the first-choice treatment for PWS lesions (Fig. 9.1a, b). Using the principle of selective photothermolysis, PDL wavelengths are absorbed by oxy- and deoxy-hemoglobin, producing heat, photocoagulation and aggregation of erythrocytes, and, ultimately, necrosis of the endothelial cells. Subsequently, intense blood vessel damage leads to either a severe reduction in or shutdown of blood flow (Heger et al. 2005). Afterwards, during the healing

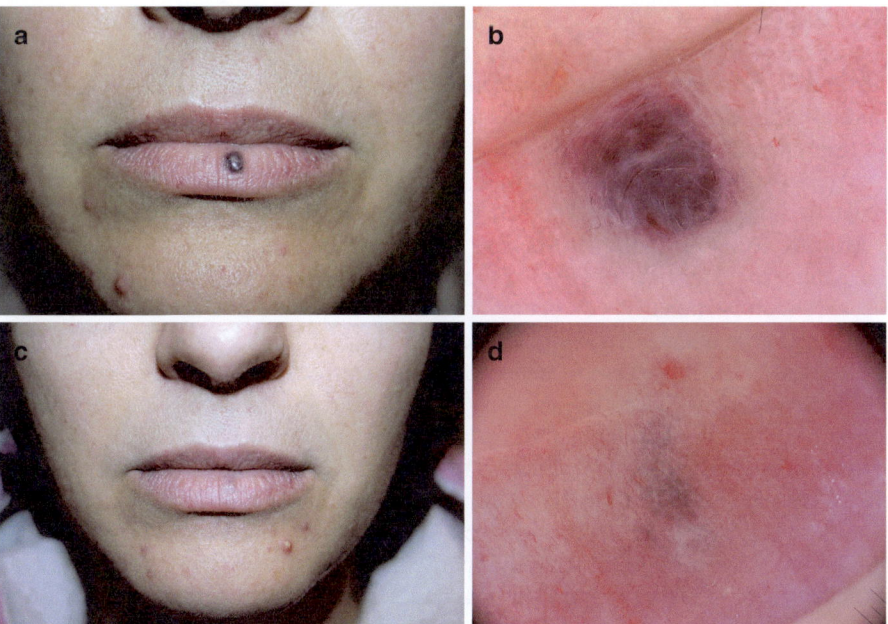

Fig. 9.1 (**a**) Clinical picture of a PWS on the lower lip in a young woman before any treatment. (**b**) Dermoscopic image of the lesion. (**c**) Clinical image after three Nd:YAG sessions. (**d**) Dermoscopic exam highlights a complete clearance of the vascular malformation due to a complete photocoagulation of the target vessels. (Courtesy of Dr. Domenico Piccolo, Skin Center Avezzano, Italy)

process, the photocoagulated vessels are replaced by normal-sized capillaries resulting in a reduction in dermal blood content and hence PWS redness (Reddy et al.
2013; Jia et al. 2010). However, in several cases, insufficiently damaged vessels can
regenerate too widely during the vascular remodeling phase based on the normal
healing response of the skin wound, and thus hinder the reduction of cutaneous
blood content (Phung et al. 2008; Jia et al. 2010). Clinically, complete photocoagulation of the target vessels is associated with a good clearance (Fiskerstrand et al.
1996a, b), representing approximately 40% of cases (Greve and Raulin 2004)
(Fig. 9.1c, d). Incomplete photocoagulation of PWS vasculature is associated with
suboptimal to no clearance, which prevails in 20–46% and 14–40% of patients,
respectively (Fiskerstrand et al. 1996a, b; Greve and Raulin 2004; Hohenleutner
et al. 1995). The reasons for such heterogeneity in PDL responses are not fully
understood. Generally, factors that reduce light penetration, such as superimposed
vasculature and high melanin content as well as an increased PWS vascular density,
diameter, or depth, may negatively affect PDL. Among these factors, vessel depth is
probably the most important character in determining the effectiveness of PWS
laser treatment. Since PDL wavelengths penetrate up to 2 mm into the skin, very
small and deep vessels are less likely to respond to PDL treatment. In addition, re-
vascularization secondary to the wound healing response after treatment may also
be an intrinsic limitation of the treatment with PDL (Phung et al. 2008). Lesion re-
darkening has been reported in 16.3–50% of patients within 5 years after PDL treatment (Michel et al. 2001; Orten et al. 1996). The effect of PDL may also be
associated with the following factors: (1) age at treatment. Younger patients show
better PDL response mainly due to thinner dermis, less epidermal melanin, and less
dermal collagen. Thus, the sooner the treatment is performed, the greater the chance
of resolving the problem.

Additionally, during their lifetime, all angiomas undergo modifications which
make the treatment more problematic. For this reason, PWS treatment in adults is
performed using much higher fluences than those used with children. This exposes
the patient to major risks of adverse events and the likelihood of therapeutic success
decreases proportionally; (2) anatomic location. Facial lesions are associated with
better response than on neck, trunk, and extremities (Sommer et al. 2003; Shi et al.
2014; Woo et al. 2006). The effects on lesions in different facial areas are also variable with central forehead lesions showing the best response followed by peripheral
facial lesions and at last by central facial lesions, and this may result from the variable skin thickness of different areas (Renfro and Geronemus 1993; Nguyen et al.
1998); (3) lesion thickness. Hypertrophy and nodularity respond poorly to PDL
treatment (Izikson et al. 2009); (4) size of PWS lesions. Smaller lesions (<20 cm^2)
are associated with better treatment response than the large ones (>40 cm^2) (Nguyen
et al. 1998); (5) number of treatments. It has been shown that patients who received
a larger number of treatments have a better laser response, with approximately 10%
improvement per treatment session (Koster et al. 2001). However, many PWSs that
initially respond well may show a diminished response to successive PDL sessions
until a plateau is reached, so that further improvement is not seen (Nguyen et al.
1998). This phenomenon may be secondary to an effect of laser treatment on vessel

morphology. Several studies have documented that prior PDL treatment results in smaller and deeper vessels post-treatment (Hohenleutner et al. 1995; Fiskerstrand et al. 1996a, b; Sivarajan and Mackay 2005). By becoming smaller, deeper vessels are more difficult to treat, thus previous treatments with a PDL may significantly contribute to resistance to subsequent treatment (Savas et al. 2013). In order to enhance PWS clearance, refractory lesions are sometimes treated with alternatives lasers and light sources, like long-pulsed 1064 nm Nd:YAG and 755 nm Alexandrite lasers and PDT, and eventually with the use of antiangiogenic drugs in combination, with the aim to produce further improvement (Izikson et al. 2009).

Short-lasting post-procedural side effects have been reported in the majority of patients and include edema, erythema, blistering, and crusting that persist for hours, and sometimes up to days or weeks. More permanent effects may also occur (Brightman et al. 2015). Pigmentary changes, such as hyperpigmentation and hypopigmentation, have been reported in 1.4% of patients, as a result of damage to melanosomes and/or post-inflammatory changes while atrophic and hypertrophic scarring have been reported in 4.3% and 0.7% of patients, respectively (Haedersdal et al. 1998; Astner and Anderson 2005).

When laser treatment is not available or when non-purpuric treatment with limited side effects is desired, intense pulsed light (IPL) may be an effective alternative to PDL for the treatment of PWSs. In a study evaluating the efficacy of IPL in 15 patients with PDL-resistant PWS, approximately half of patients obtained more than 50% reduction of their lesions (Bjerring et al. 2003). In another study of 30 patients with previously untreated PWS, it was found that 100% of patients showed more than 25% clearance, while 30% of patients were able to achieve 75% clearance (Dong et al. 2010). Babilas and colleagues (2010) conducted a split-face study using IPL and PDL and found that an IPL with a wavelength range of 555–950 nm achieved better outcomes than the PDL ($\lambda = 585$ nm). On the other hand, in another head-to-head study, Faurschou et al. (2009) evaluated 20 patients with PWS and found that both PDL and IPL lightened PWS, but the median clinical improvement was significantly better for PDL (65%) than IPL (30%). Nevertheless, IPL, under certain treatment parameters, has the potential to be an effective treatment for PWS clearance both in terms of a reduction in the number of treatments and improved efficiency of each treatment, especially for these lesions which do not respond to PDL therapy.

In this chapter, many selected PWSs were treated with IPL. The choice of IPL was based on its variability of pulse and fluence and its possibility to divide the energy into different pulses, allowing an additional heating which leads to coagulation of blood vessels of different diameter and different depth (Piccolo et al. 2014). A 500 nm filter (46×10 mm) was used. Two pulses of 5 ms and 10 ms, respectively, were used with a delay of 10 ms. The fluency selected was a determining factor for the results and varied between 14 and 17 J/cm^2, with two or three consecutive passages. IPL systems require considerable experience and should be conducted with the aid of a good dermoscopy in order to determine the type of vessels to treat (Piccolo 2012; Piccolo 2014).

9.2   The Validity of Dermoscopy in the Treatment of Flat Angiomas and PWS

On dermoscopy, PWSs are characterized by two main microvascular patterns which correlate with their histology: (1) a superficial or blob pattern (Type 1) consisting of red globules and dots that correspond to dilated, capillary loops in the papillary dermis, and (2) a deep pattern (Type 2) with red ring structures corresponding to dilated vessels located deep in the horizontal vascular plexus (Motley et al. 1997; Eubanks and McBurney 2001; Procaccini et al. 2001; Haliasos et al. 2013). Recently, Procaccini et al. (2001) proposed another pattern consisting of a gray-whitish veil whose presence is linked to deep PWSs. In addition, Sevila et al. (2004) observed two other dermoscopic findings: (1) an undefined pattern consisting of a complete absence of any of the previously reported patterns and the presence of streaks of white linear structures with a rose, whitish, or blue background; (2) a pale halo surrounding a central brownish dot.

According to the literature, there is a close correlation between the patterns and features observed dermoscopically and the anatomic areas of PWSs. Eubacks and McBurney (2001) reported that lesions located at the third branch of the trigeminal nerve, neck, and thorax were more likely to have a superficial type 1 pattern while those located at the second branch of the trigeminal nerve and distal extremities were more likely to have a deeper type 2 pattern. In contrast, Sevila (Sevila et al. 2004) did not find statistically significant differences in the pattern as related to the involved trigeminal branch, but instead to centrofacial vs. peripheral distribution.

The dermoscopic exam performed before treatment efficaciously highlights the number and gauge, but also the depth of the vessels to be treated (Figs. 9.2a, b, 9.3a, b, 9.4a, b, and 9.5a, b).

The vessels targeted are the more superficial ones which will therefore better respond to treatment. The dermoscopic exam performed immediately after treatment reveals the color change from red to blue (Figs. 9.2c, d, 9.3c, d, 9.4c, d, and 9.5c, d).

The greater the number of vessels hit, the greater the risk of consequential damage on the days immediately after treatment, thus leading to the formation of erosions and scabs. However, the presence of scabs does not influence the final results: usually, the areas most intensively treated are those that will present the best final results.

In the areas where vessels persist, more than one session may be necessary as it is possible that vessels which resisted in the first treatment will disappear in the following session. This gives excellent clinical results (Figs. 9.2e, f, 9.5c, d, and 9.6a, b).

Recently, vascular filters are provided with some picture analysis software tools so that both clinicians and patients can easily verify the efficacy of laser treatment (Figs. 9.6c, 9.7a, b, and 9.8a, b).

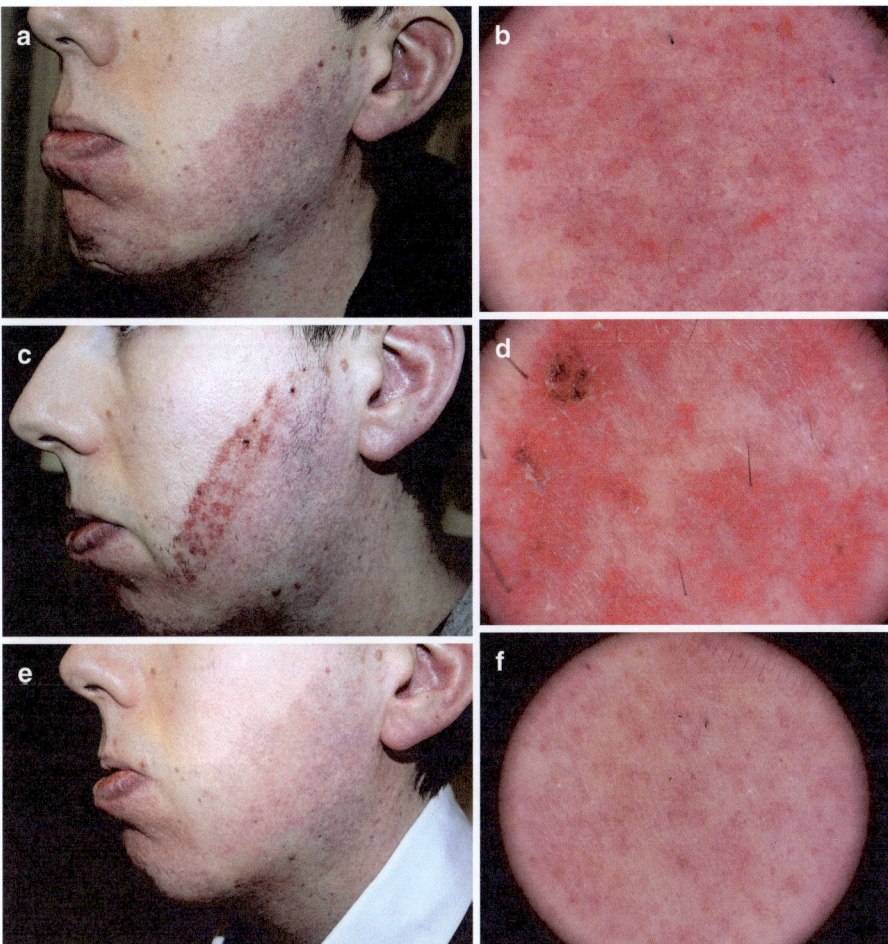

Fig. 9.2 (**a**) Clinical picture of a flat angioma on the cheek in a young man before any treatment. (**b**) Dermoscopy performed before any treatment is useful to highlight the number and gauge, but also the depth of the vessels to be treated. (**c**) Clinical image taken immediately after treatment. (**d**) The dermoscopic exam performed immediately after treatment reveals the color change from red to blue. In the areas where vessels persist, more than one session may be necessary as it is possible that vessels which resisted in the first treatment will disappear in the following session. (**e**) Clinical image after three dye laser sessions. (**f**) The excellent clinical results are confirmed at the dermoscopy. (Courtesy of Dr. Domenico Piccolo, Skin Center Avezzano, Italy)

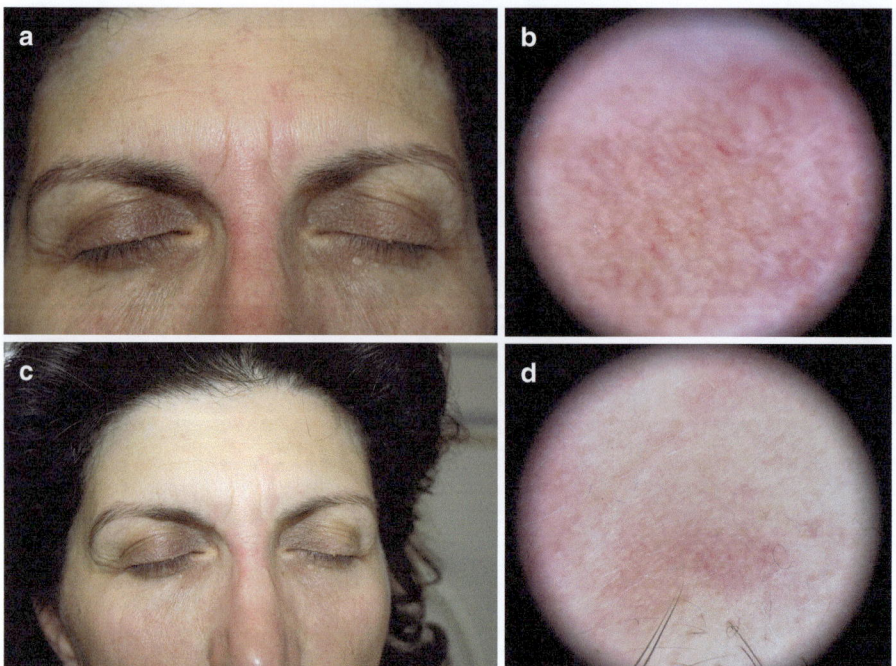

Fig. 9.3 (**a**) Clinical picture of a PWS on the nose and glabella in a woman before any treatment. (**b**) Dermoscopy image of the lesion highlights the increased number of small vessels. (**c**) Clinical image after three Nd:YAG sessions. (**d**) Dermoscopic exam highlights a complete clearance of the vascular malformation due to a complete photocoagulation of the target vessels. (Courtesy of Dr. Domenico Piccolo, Skin Center Avezzano, Italy)

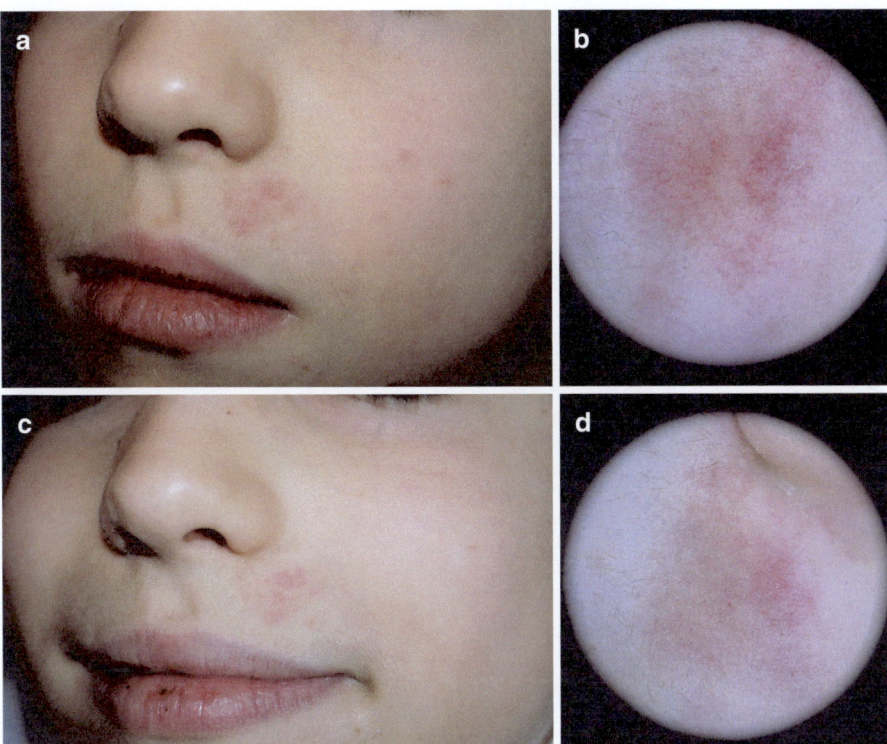

Fig. 9.4 (**a**) Clinical picture of a flat angioma sited on the upper lip in a child before any treatment. (**b**) Dermoscopy image of the lesion highlights the increased number of small vessels. (**c**) Clinical image after two Nd:YAG sessions. (**d**) Dermoscopic exam highlights a complete clearance of the lesion. (Courtesy of Dr. Domenico Piccolo, Skin Center Avezzano, Italy)

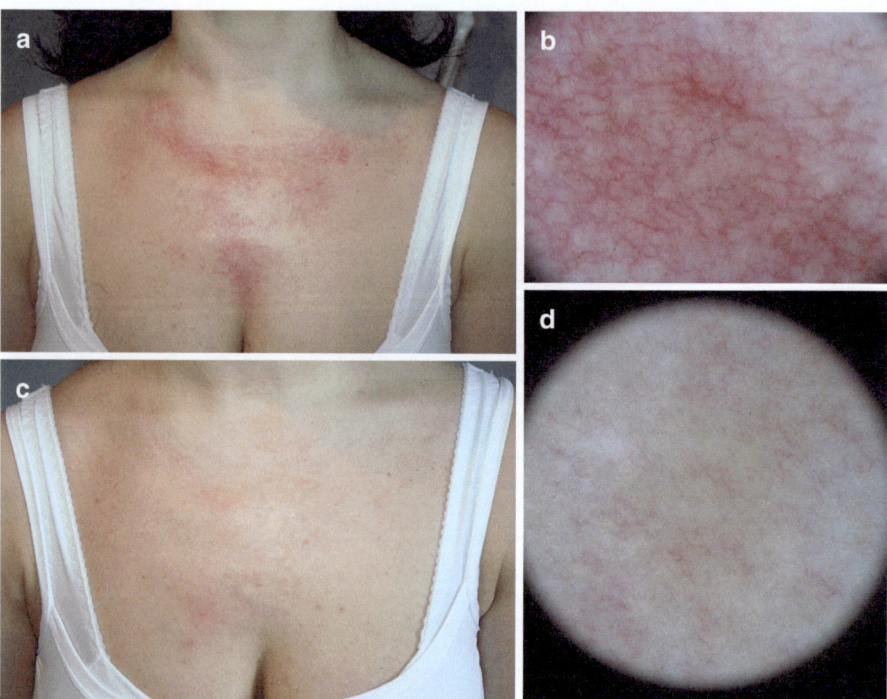

Fig. 9.5 (**a**) Clinical picture of a PWS of the décolleté in a young woman before any treatment. (**b**) Dermoscopy image of the lesion highlights the increased number of small vessels. (**c**) Clinical image after three Nd:YAG sessions. (**d**) Dermoscopic exam highlights a complete clearance of the vascular malformation due to a complete photocoagulation of the target vessels. (Courtesy of Dr. Domenico Piccolo, Skin Center Avezzano, Italy)

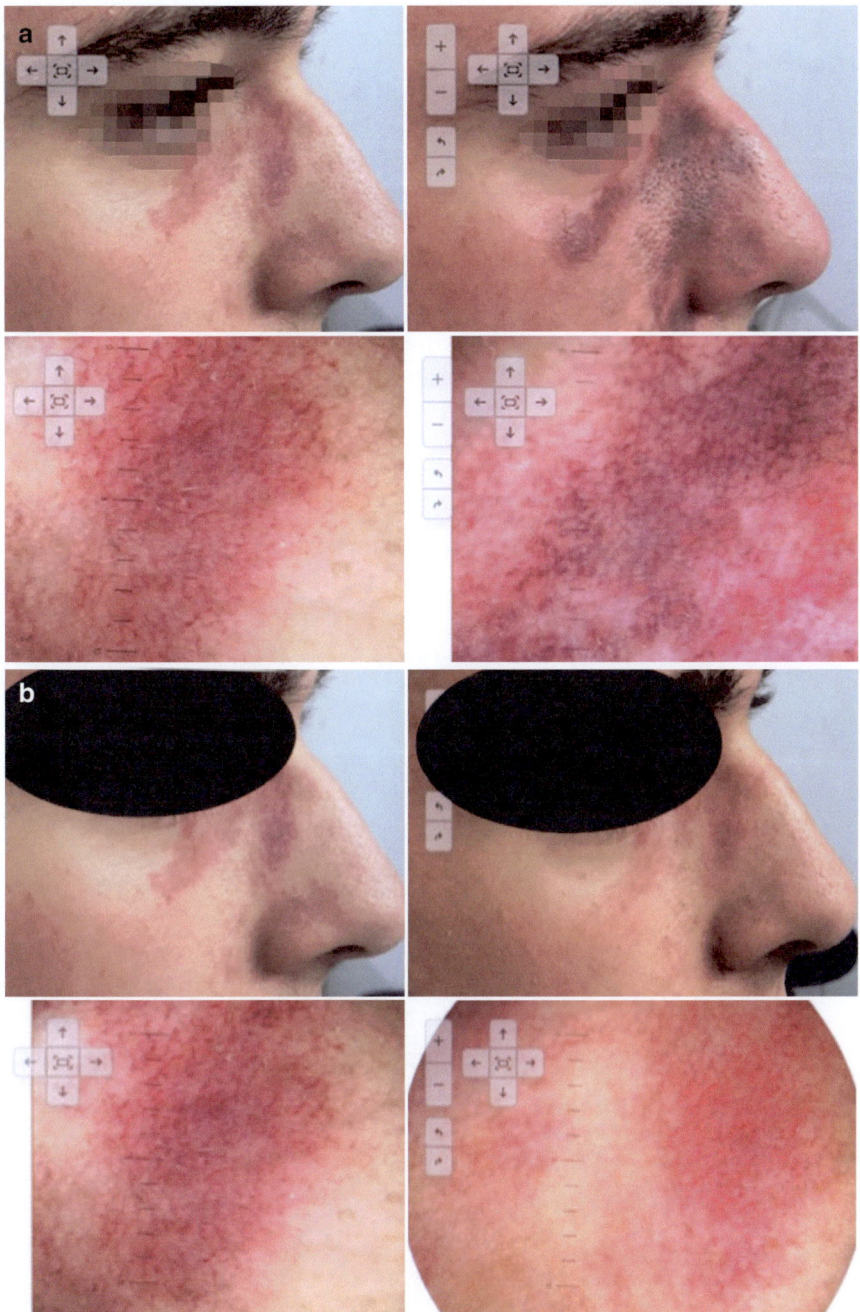

Fig. 9.6 (**a**) Clinical and dermoscopic picture of a facial angioma in a young man before any treatment and immediately after one dye laser session. (**b**) Clinical and dermoscopic picture before any treatment and immediately after 48 days from the dye laser session. (**c**) The software's vascular filter highlights a significant reduction in the angiomatous component. (Courtesy of Dr. Domenico Piccolo, Skin Center Avezzano, Italy)

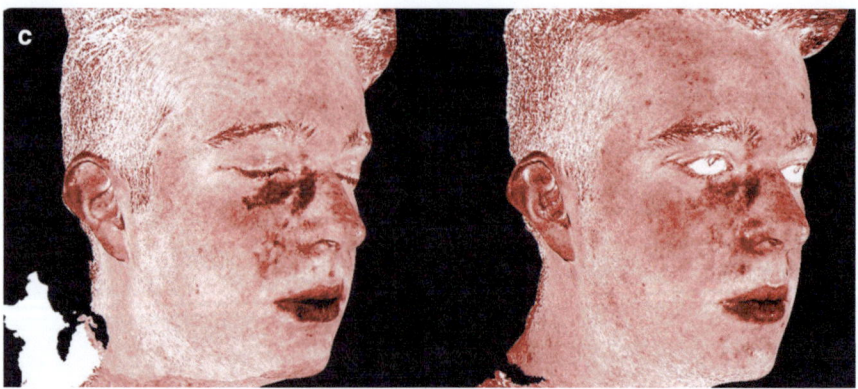

Fig. 9.6 (continued)

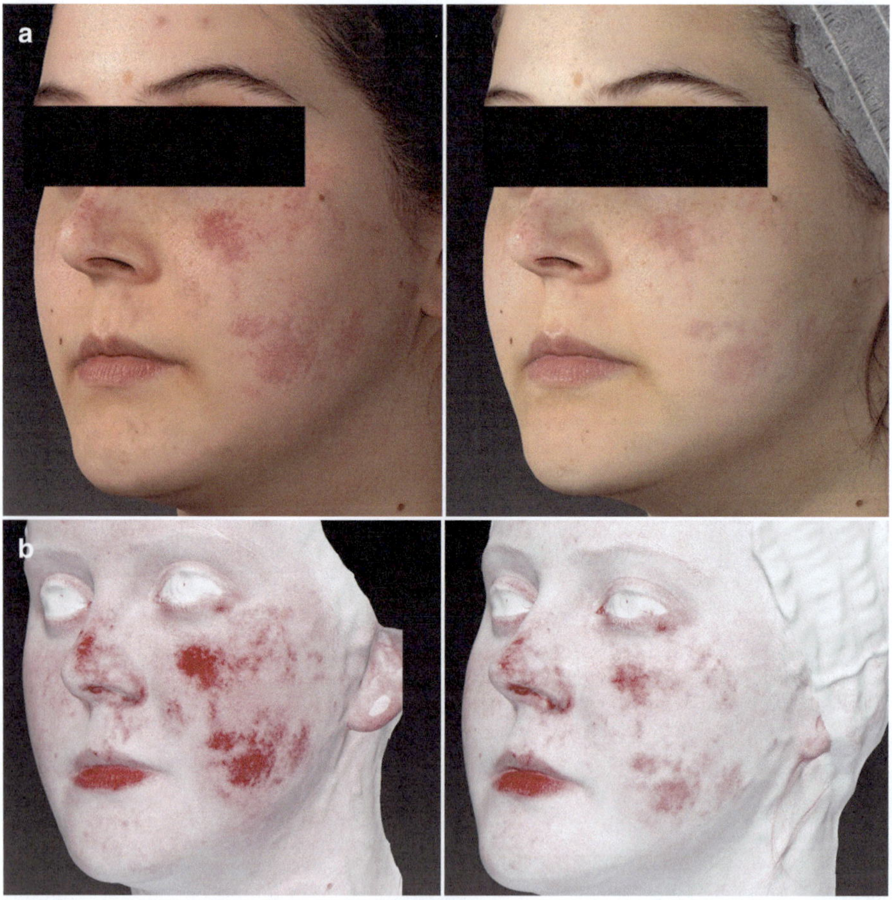

Fig. 9.7 (**a**) Clinical picture of a facial angioma in a young woman before any treatment and immediately after three dye laser session. (**b**) The software's vascular filter highlights a significant reduction in the vascular component. (Courtesy of Dr. Domenico Piccolo, Skin Center Avezzano, Italy)

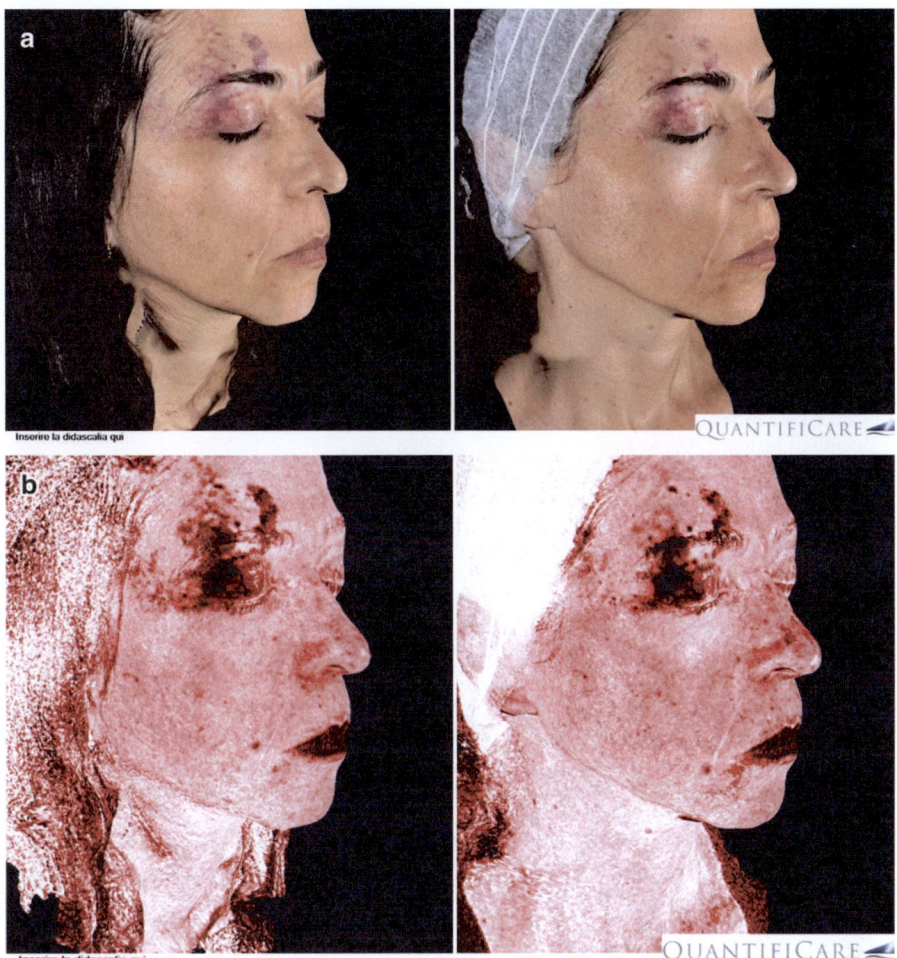

Fig. 9.8 (**a**) Clinical picture of a periocular angioma in a young woman before any treatment and immediately after three dye laser session. (**b**) The software's vascular filter highlights a significant reduction in the vascular component. (Courtesy of Dr. Domenico Piccolo, Skin Center Avezzano, Italy)

References

Adams BB, Lucky AW. Acquired portwine stains and antecedent trauma: case report and review of the literature. Arch Dermatol. 2000;136:897–9.

Astner S, Anderson RR. Treating vascular lesions. Dermatol Ther. 2005;18:267–81.

Babilas P, Schreml S, Eames T, et al. Split-face comparison of intense pulsed light with short- and long-pulsed dye lasers for the treatment of port-wine stains. Lasers Surg Med. 2010;42:720–7.

Bansal S, Garg VK, Wadhwa B, et al. Acquired port-wine stain in an adult male: first reported case from India with review of literature. Indian J Dermatol. 2015;60:104.

Barsky SH, Rosen S, Geer DE, et al. The Nature and Evolution of Port Wine Stains: A Computer-assisted Study. J Invest Dermatol. 1980;74(3):154–57.

Bjerring P, Christiansen K, Troilius A. Intense pulsed light source for the treatment of dye laser resistant port-wine stains. J Cosmet Laser Ther. 2003;5:7–13.

Brightman LA, Geronemus RG, Reddy KK. Laser treatment of port-wine stains. Clin Cosmet Investig Dermatol. 2015;8:27–33.

Burns AJ, Navarro JA. Role of laser therapy in pediatric patients. Plast Reconstr Surg. 2009;124(1 Suppl):82e–92e.

Chen JK, Ghasri P, Aguilar G, et al. An overview of clinical and experimental treatment modalities for port wine stains. J Am Acad Dermatol. 2012;67:289–304.

Colver GB, Ryan TJ. Acquired port-wine stain. Arch Dermatol. 1986;122:1415–6.

Dong X, Yu Q, Ding J, et al. Treatment of facial port-wine stains with a new intense pulsed light source in Chinese patients. J Cosmet Laser Ther. 2010;12:183–7.

van Drooge AM, Beek JF, van der Veen JP, et al. Hypertrophy in port-wine stains: prevalence and patient characteristics in a large patient cohort. J Am Acad Dermatol. 2012;67:1214–9.

Enjolras O, Riche MC, Merland JJ. Facial port-wine stains and Sturge-Weber syndrome. Pediatrics. 1985;76:48–51.

Eubanks LE, McBurney EI. Videomicroscopy of port-wine stains: correlation of location and depth of lesion. J Am Acad Dermatol. 2001;44:948–51.

Faurschou A, Togsverd-Bo K, Zachariae C, et al. Pulsed dye laser vs. intense pulsed light for port-wine stains: a randomized side-by-side trial with blinded response evaluation. Br J Dermatol. 2009;160:359–64.

Finley JL, Noe JM, Arndt KA, et al. Port-wine stains. Morphologic variations and developmental lesions. Arch Dermatol. 1984;120:1453–5.

Fiskerstrand EJ, Svaasand LO, Kopstad G, et al. Laser treatment of port wine stains: therapeutic outcome in relation to morphological parameters. Br J Dermatol. 1996a;134:1039–43.

Fiskerstrand EJ, Svaasand LO, Kopstad G, et al. Photothermally induced vessel-wall necrosis after pulsed dye laser treatment: lack of response in port-wine stains with small sized or deeply located vessels. J Invest Dermatol. 1996b;107:671–5.

Freysz M, Cribier B, Lipsker D. Fegelers syndrome, acquired port-wine stain or acquired capillary malformation: three cases and a literature review. Ann Dermatol Venereol. 2013;140:341–6.

Geronemus RG, Ashinoff R. The medical necessity of evaluation and treatment of port- wine stains. J Dermatol Surg Oncol. 1991;17:76–9.

Greve B, Raulin C. Prospective study of port wine stain treatment with dye laser: comparison of two wavelengths (585 nm vs 595 nm) and two pulse durations (0.5 milliseconds vs 20 milliseconds). Lasers Surg Med. 2004;34:168–73.

Haedersdal M, Gniadecka M, Efsen J, et al. Side effects from the pulsed dye laser: the importance of skin pigmentation and skin redness. Acta Derm Venereol. 1998;78:445–50.

Hagen SL, Grey KR, Korta DZ, et al. Quality of life in adults with facial port-wine stains. J Am Acad Dermatol. 2017;76(4):695–702.

Haliasos EC, Kerner M, Jaimes N, et al. Dermoscopy for the pediatric dermatologist, part ii: dermoscopy of genetic syndromes with cutaneous manifestations and pediatric vascular lesions. Pediatr Dermatol. 2013;30:172–81.

Heger M, Beek JF, Moldovan NI, et al. Towards optimization of selective photothermolysis: prothrombotic pharmaceutical agents as potential adjuvants in laser treatment of port wine stains. A theoretical study. Thromb Haemost. 2005;93:242–56.

Hershkovitz D, Bercovich D, Sprecher E, et al. RASA1 mutations may cause hereditary capillary malformations without arteriovenous malformations. Br J Dermatol. 2008;158:1035–40.

Hohenleutner U, Hilbert M, Wlotzke U, et al. Epidermal damage and limited coagulation depth with the flashlamp-pumped pulsed dye laser: a histochemical study. J Invest Dermatol. 1995;104:798–802.

Hoque S, Holden C. Acquired port wine stain following oral isotretinoin. Clin Exp Dermatol. 2005;30:587–8.

van der Horst CM, de Borgie CA, et al. Psychosocial adjustment of children and adults with port wine stains. Br J Plast Surg. 1997;50:463–7.

Izikson L, Nelson JS, Anderson RR. Treatment of hypertrophic and resistant port wine stains with a 755 nm laser: a case series of 20 patients. Lasers Surg Med. 2009;41:427–32.

Jacobs AH, Walton RG. The incidence of birthmarks in the neonate. Pediatrics. 1976;58:218–22.

Jia W, Sun V, Tran N, et al. Long-term blood vessel removal with combined laser and topical rapamycin antiangiogenic therapy: implications for effective port wine stain treatment. Lasers Surg Med. 2010;42:105–12.

Klapman MH, Yao JF. Thickening and nodules in port-wine stains. J Am Acad Dermatol. 2001;44:300–2.

Koster PHL, van der Horst CMAM, van Gemert MJC, et al. Histologic evaluation of skin damage after overlapping and nonoverlapping flashlamp pumped pulsed dye laser pulses: A study on normal human skin as a model for port wine stains. Laser Surg Med. 2001;28(2):176–81.

Lanigan SW, Cotterill JA. Psychological disabilities amongst patients with port wine stains. Br J Dermatol. 1989;121:209–15.

Lanigan SW, Cotterill JA. Reduced vasoactive responses in port wine stains. Br J Dermatol. 1990;122:615–22.

Li G, Lin T, Wu Q, et al. Clinical analysis of port wine stains treated by intense pulsed light. J Cosmet Laser Ther. 2010;12:2–6.

Malm M, Carlberg M. Port-wine stain--a surgical and psychological problem. Ann Plast Surg. 1988;20:512–6.

Masnari O, Schiestl C, Rössler J, et al. Stigmatization predicts psychological adjustment and quality of life in children and adolescents with a facial difference. J Pediatr Psychol. 2013;38:162–72.

Michel S, Landthaler M, Hohenleutner U. Recurrence of port-wine stains after treatment with the flashlamp-pumped pulsed dye laser. Br J Dermatol. 2001;143(6):1230–34.

Motley RJ, Lanigan SW, Katugampola GA. Videomicroscopy predicts outcome in treatment of port-wine stains. Arch Dermatol. 1997;133:921–2.

Nguyen CM, Yohn JJ, Huff C, et al. Facial port wine stains in childhood: prediction of the rate of improvement as a function of the age of the patient, size and location of the port wine stain and the number of treatments with the pulsed dye (585 nm) laser. Br J Dermatol. 1998;138:821–5.

Orten SS, Waner M, Flock S, et al. Port-wine Stains: An Assessment of 5 Years of Treatment. Archives of Otolaryngology - Head and Neck Surgery. 1996;122(11):1174–79.

Osburn K, Schosser RH, Everett MA. Congenital pigmented and vascular lesions in newborn infants. J Am Acad Dermatol. 1987;16:788–92.

Phung TL, Oble DA, Jia W, Benjamin LE, et al. Can the wound healing response of human skin be modulated after laser treatment and the effects of exposure extended? Implications on the combined use of the pulsed dye laser and a topical angiogenesis inhibitor for treatment of port wine stain birthmarks. Lasers Surg Med. 2008;40:1–5.

Piccolo D. The usefulness of dermoscopy in laser and intense pulsed light treatments. Remo Sandron: Florence; 2012.

Piccolo D, Di Marcantonio D, Crisman G, et al. Unconventional use of intense pulsed light. Biomed Res Int. 2014;2014:618206.

Procaccini EM, Argenziano G, Staibano S, et al. Epiluminescence microscopy for port- wine stains: pretreatment evaluation. Dermatology. 2001;203:329.

Rajan N, Ryan J, Langtry JAA. Squamous Cell Carcinoma Arising Within a Facial Port-Wine Stain Treated by Mohs Micrographic Surgical Excision. Dermatol Surg. 2006;32(6):864–66.

Reddy KK, Brauer JA, Idriss MH, et al. Treatment of port-wine stains with a short pulse width 532-nm Nd:YAG laser. J Drugs Dermatol. 2013;12:66–71.

Renfro L, Geronemus RG. Anatomical differences of port wine stains in response to treatment with the pulsed dye laser. Arch Dermatol. 1993;129:182–8.

Rosen S, Smoller B. Pathogenesis of port wine stains. A new hypothesis. Med Hypotheses. 1987;22:365–8.

Salim A, Kurwa H, Turner R. Acquired port-wine stain associated with glaucoma. Clin Exp Dermatol. 2003;28:230–1.

Savas JA, Ledon JA, Franca K, et al. Pulsed dye laser-resistant port-wine stains: mechanisms of resistance and implications for treatment. Br J Dermatol. 2013;168:941–53.

Senti G, Trüeb RM. Acquired naevus flammeus (Fegeler syndrome). Vasa. 2000;29:225–8.

Sevila A, Nagore E, Botella-Estrada R, et al. Videomicroscopy of Venular Malformations (Port-Wine Stain Type): Prediction of Response to Pulsed Dye Laser. Pediatr Dermatol. 2004;21(5):589–96.

Sheehan DJ, Lesher JL Jr. Pyogenic granuloma arising within a Port-Wine Stain. Cutis. 2004;73(3):175–80.

Shi W, Wang J, Lin Y, et al. Treatment of port wine stains with pulsed dye laser: a retrospective study of 848 cases in Shandong Province, People's Republic of China. Drug Des Devel Ther. 2014;8:2531–82014.

Silapunt S, Goldberg LH, Thurber M, et al. Basal cell carcinoma arising in a port-wine stain. Dermatol Surg. 2004;30:1241–5.

Sivarajan V, Mackay IR. Noninvasive in vivo assessment of vessel characteristics in capillary vascular malformations exposed to five pulsed dye laser treatments. Plast Reconstr Surg. 2005;115:1245–52.

Sommer S, Seukeran DC, Sheehan-Dare RA. Efficacy of pulsed dye laser treatment of port wine stain malformations of the lower limb. Br J Dermatol. 2003;149:770–5.

Vural E, Ramakrishnan J, Cetin N, et al. The expression of vascular endothelial growth factor and its receptors in port-wine stains. Otolaryngol Head Neck Surg. 2008;139:560–4.

Woo SH, Ahn HH, Kim SN, et al. Treatment of vascular skin lesions with the variable-pulse 595 nm pulsed dye laser. Dermatol Surg. 2006;32:41–8.

Wu Y, Yu RJ, Chen D, et al. Glaucoma in patients with eyes close to areas affected by port-wine stain has lateral and gender predilection. Chin Med J. 2017;130:2922–6.

Dermoscopy Applied to Laser and IPL Treatments: Acne and Post-traumatic Scars

10

Acne is a chronic inflammatory disease of the pilosebaceous unit clinically characterized by the presence of comedones, inflammatory papules, pustules, and sometimes nodules and cysts. Acne is estimated to affect 9.4% of the global population, making it the eighth most prevalent disease worldwide (Tan and Bhate 2015). Epidemiological studies have demonstrated that acne affects nearly 80% of young people aged 12–25 years (Kraning and Odland 1979; James 2005). Although more common in post-pubescent adolescents, with boys more frequently affected, particularly with more severe forms of the disease (Ghodsi et al. 2009), about 20–40% of cases persist until the fourth and fifth decade (persistent acne) or it also has its initial onset in old age (late-onset acne) (Gollnick and Zouboulis 2014; Degitz and Ochsendorf 2017).

Acne pathogenesis is attributed to multiple factors such as hyperseborrhoea, abnormal follicular keratinization, alteration of the quality of sebum lipids, androgen activity, proliferation of *Propionibacterium acnes*, and production of perifollicular inflammation (Layton 2001; Degitz et al. 2007). In addition, various physiological and exogenous factors act as triggers or modulators, including androgens, growth factors (i.e., IGF-1), neuroendocrine mediators, drugs, and Western dietary habits (foods with a high glycemic load, dairy products) (Gollnick 2015; Moradi Tuchayi et al. 2015). In some patients, the severe inflammatory response to *Propionibacterium acnes* results in permanent, disfiguring scars.

Overall prevalence of acne scarring has yet to be entirely clarified. In a French population analysis, a validated self-administered questionnaire was used to identify cases of acne sequelae among 3305 women aged 25–40 years. The scar prevalence in that analysis was observed to be 49% (Poli et al. 2001). A similar scar prevalence of 52.6% has been found in another self-reported survey conducted among adolescents in Hong Kong (Yeung et al. 2002). Goulden et al. (1999) examined 231 women and 130 men aged over 25 years for facial acne and found a scar

The contents of this book are partially based on the Italian language edition: "*The Usefulness of Dermoscopy in Laser and IPL Treatments*", Domenico Piccolo, © DEKA M.E.L.A Srl 2012.

© Springer Nature Switzerland AG 2020

D. Piccolo et al., *Quick Guide to Dermoscopy in Laser and IPL Treatments*, https://doi.org/10.1007/978-3-319-41633-5_10

prevalence of 11% in males and 14% in females. Kilkenny et al. (1998) reported a scar prevalence of 26.1% among 266 Australian school students aged 16–18. Likewise, in another study conducted by Lauermann et al. (2016) out of 2201 male adolescents aged 18 years, 22% exhibited acne scarring.

The pathogenesis of atrophic scars is not fully understood. It is most likely related to inflammatory mediators and enzymatic degradation of collagen fibers and subcutaneous fat (Fife 2011). The propensity to develop scars varies among individuals, and apparently depends on individually different immunological responses during the first phase of healing (Holland et al. 2004; Saint-Jean et al. 2016). Holland et al. (2004) showed that in patients prone to scarring, early lesions have a large, active nonspecific inflammatory response which subsided in resolution lesions. In contrast, in patients not prone to scarring, early lesions have smaller, more specific immune response that was increased and activated in resolving lesions, suggesting that this excessive and prolonged immune response may contribute to scarring.

Although scarring has been reported to predominantly occur in patients with severe acne (Lauermann et al. 2016), the degree of acne does not always correlate with the incidence or severity of scarring. In a recent study of 1972 subjects with acne, 43% had acne scarring. Among these, subjects with acne scars were significantly more likely to have severe or very severe acne ($p < 0.01$); however, 69% of those with acne scars had mild or moderate acne at the time of the study visit (Tan et al. 2017a, b). Likewise, Hayashi et al. (2015) reported that patients with scars experienced significantly more severe acne symptoms than patients without scars ($p = 0.025$), although 15.0% of patients with scars had experienced only mild acne symptoms. These results indicate that scarring may occur with even milder acne forms. Delayed treatment and duration of acne may also be associated with the extent and severity of scarring. Layton et al. (1994) showed that, after a 3-year mean acne duration, up to 95% of individuals experienced some degree of facial scarring. Other risk factors of scarring include genetic factors, ineffective inflammatory response, onset of acne at young age, frequent relapses, truncal localization, and ethnicity (Tan et al. 2017a, b).

It is important to recognize that scarring is sequelae of an individual lesion and thus can occur in any stage of acne. Almost all acne scars generally arise from post-inflammatory lesions including macular erythema (83%), and only some (16%) from inflammatory acne lesions such as papules and pustules (Tan et al. 2017a, b). In addition, scarring may be the consequence of squeezing or picking lesions with the fingernails. Once scarring has occurred, it is usually permanent and often worsens over time, mainly due to the normal effects of aging (O'Daniel 2011).

There are two basic types of scar based on whether there is an aberrant production or degradation of collagen, with differing pathogenesis and clinical management. As many as 80–90% of patients with acne scars have so-called atrophic scars, or scars associated with a net loss of collagen in the dermis, while only 10–20% of these patients develop hypertrophic scars or keloids (due to an exuberance of collagen production in the healing process). In addition to collagen variations, these scars can be erythematous, hyperpigmented, and/or hypopigmented as acne scars can be accentuated by post-inflammatory erythema (PIE) and/or post-inflammatory hyperpigmentation (PIH). PIE refers to localized skin erythema resulting from microvascular dilation related to wound healing, most commonly present in lighter skin types (I–III) (Bae-Harboe and Graber 2013). On the other hand, PIH describes subsequent pigment change and it is typically seen in darker skin types (IV–VI) (Davis and Callender 2010). PIH may result from the overproduction of melanin or an irregular dispersion of pigment after cutaneous inflammation as well as after aggressive treatments for acne (Stratigos and Katsambas 2004).

According to the literature, many instruments have been proposed to evaluate the severity of acne scar, particularly the atrophic ones (Fife 2011; Fabbrocini et al. 2010), but to date no scale has been generally accepted to estimate the gravity and the psycho-emotional effect deriving from it. The most basic, practical and widespread classification among experts was created by Jacob (2001) and includes three types of atrophic scars according to scar morphology: (1) icepick scars (60–70%), defined as narrow, less-than-2 mm, V-shaped epithelial tracts, sharply marginated that extend vertically to the deep dermis or subcutaneous tissue; (2) boxcar scars (20–30%), defined as depressed lesions of 1.5–4.0 mm in diameter, round-to-oval with sharply demarcated vertical edges, which are clinically wider at the surface than icepick scars and do not taper to a point at the basis, and they can also be distinguished in shallow (0.1–0.5 mm) or deep (≥0.5 mm); (3) rolling scars (15–25%), which are the widest and may reach up to 5 mm in diameter.

It is important to note that sometimes different types of scars can be observed in the same patient making differentiation difficult.

The Europeans acne group (ECCA) has renamed the atrophic acne scars as V-shaped (icepick), U-shaped (boxcar), and W-shaped (rolling) (Dreno et al. 2007). Goodman and Baron proposed a qualitative scale and then presented a quantitative scale. Their system relies on a scar count by type, calculating a score according to the number and severity of each type which vary from a minimum of 0 to a maximum of 84 points (Goodman and Baron 2006). Others acne scar severity grading scales include Vancouver Scar Scale (VSS), Patient and Observer Scar Assessment Scale (POSAS), Visual Analog Scale (VAS), and the Patient Satisfaction Score (PSS) (Fearmonti et al. 2010). The most common anatomical area affected by acne scar is the face (55% of subjects), followed by the back (24%) and chest (14%) (Tan et al. 2017a, b). On the face, atrophic scarring is most frequent on malar region (80%), forehead (31.5%), mentonian region (16.5%), and nose (Lauermann et al. 2016).

Acne scarring may cause substantial physical and psychological distress, particularly in adolescents, associated with poor self-esteem, depression, anxiety, altered social interactions, body image alterations, embarrassment, anger, lower academic performance, and unemployment (Koo and Smith 1991; Koo 1995; Cotterill and Cunliffe 1997). Given the negative impact on patient quality, prevention and early initiation of an effective therapy to avoid acne scars are recommended (Hayashi et al. 2015). It is important to determine which patients are at increased risk of scarring so that they can be identified with the goal of establishing effective acne therapy.

10.1   Treatment Options

Nowadays, the treatment of the acne scar remains a challenge, mainly due to the variability of the scars, in terms of type, depth, and extension, in each individual patient, thus guaranteeing a personalized therapy, with different scars that require different therapeutic approaches (Goodman 2003; O'Daniel 2011). Furthermore, the variation of assessment tools and the lack of standardization of clinical trials make it difficult to compare treatment options. Finally, aging can accentuate the appearance of acne scars since aging is characterized by collagen and fat loss as well as the acne scars (O'Daniel 2011). The complete resolution of acne scars has not been achieved since many of the existing treatments present uncertain efficacy, potential risk of side effects (infection, hyperpigmentation, prolonged erythema, swelling), and substantial recovery times. Before starting any procedure, active acne should have been treated as new acne breakouts can lead to new acne scars. Treatment should initially be focused on erythema, if present, and then on dealing with acne scars based on the type and degree of atrophic scarring present (Connolly et al. 2017).

In clinical practice, a multimodal approach to scar treatment is usually required to achieve significant improvement given the variable morphology of acne scars, especially when more types of scars are found in the same patient. Other factors that should be taken into consideration before the start of treatment include the patient's baseline skin phototype, patient preferences, side effects, costs, patient expectations, and treatment availability.

In recent decades, numerous treatments have been proposed to mitigate this severe skin imperfections with varying degrees of efficacy and safety. Chemical peeling (Clark and Scerri 2008), dermabrasion (Fernandes et al. 2014), punch techniques (Grevelink and White 1998), subcision (Orentreich and Orentreich 1995), fat transplantation (Goodman 2003), dermal fillers (Hirsch and Cohen 2006), and needling (Fife 2011) have been used but with suboptimal outcomes (Gozali and Zhou 2015).

With the developments in laser technology, significant clinical improvements have been reported with ablative lasers such as carbon dioxide (CO_2) and Erbium:yttrium-aluminum-garnet lasers (Er:YAG). However, side effects, including infection, hyperpigmentation and discomfort, along with the long recovery time have limited their widespread use. To overcome these limitations, nonablative lasers such as diodes, Neodymium-doped yttrium aluminum garnet (Nd:YAG), and pulsed dye lasers have been used for the treatment of acne scars, with minimal downtime and side effects, but with lower clinical effects than ablative lasers.

The low safety profile of ablative lasers and the modest efficacy results of nonablative lasers led to the introduction of fractional lasers and radiofrequency (RF) technologies. Fractional lasers are based on the well-established concept of fractional damage, namely fractional photothermolysis (FP), which enables rapid post-procedural re-epithelialization through the help of the intervening skin which remains intact for the reparative process (Manstein et al. 2004; Pavlidis and Katsambas 2017). In technical terms, these devices generate thermal injury columns of controlled diameter and depth that extend through the epidermis into the dermis, called microthermal zones (MTZs), alternated with healthy tissue (Manstein et al. 2004). These areas can be either nonablative or ablative according to the device used.

Several studies have shown that fractional lasers can improve the appearance of acne scars with a good safety profile and good patient satisfaction (Alster et al. 2007; Walgrave et al. 2009; Mahmoud et al. 2010; Manuskiatti et al. 2010; Chan et al. 2010). Compared to nonablative devices, greater efficacy in the improvement of acne scars can be achieved by fractional ablative lasers, mainly due to the deep vaporization of the tissues as well as a significant coagulative effect (Elsaie et al. 2018; You et al. 2016; Cho et al. 2010). On the other hand, nonablative fractional lasers allow to obtain good results with less pain and less post-treatment recovery time, since the stratum corneum remains intact and the epidermal barrier function is preserved after treatment (Elsaie et al. 2018). Among fractional ablative devices, laser CO_2 is considered to be the best at treating acne scars (Reinholz et al. 2015) with an average improvement level of 66.8% (Chapas et al. 2008).

To improve therapeutic efficacy, recently the fractional CO_2 laser has been combined with the simultaneous use of bipolar radiofrequency without increasing the side effects (Tenna et al. 2012; Gotkin and Sarnoff 2014; Cannarozzo et al. 2014). A pilot study was conducted to evaluate the clinical efficacy of the Smartxide2 DOT/radiofrequency (RF) device (DEKA, Calenzano, Italy) on 15 subjects suffering from acne scars. Clinical evaluation using a global aesthetic improvement scale showed that 73.3% of patients were much improved or better immediately after their last treatment with 100% seeing an improvement at 12 months follow-up (Tenna et al. 2012). In a larger study of 79 patients, Campolmi et al. (2013) demonstrated that the CO_2 laser combined with the radiofrequency device is effective in the treatment of various dermatological, surgical, and aesthetic fields, including scarring and facial photoaging, and it can also be used in the treatment of traumatic scars (i.e., domestic or road accidents).

10.2   The Validity of Dermoscopy in the Treatment of Acne and Post-traumatic Scars

The use of dermoscopy has also been shown to be extremely significant in the treatment of acne scars or accident scars. Dermoscopy helps determine the depth of the scar before treatment, demonstrating the results of the treatments and ascertaining whether the use of bipolar radiofrequency was able to further improve the aesthetic result.

Therefore, we herein report on ten patients (six females and four males) with facial acne scars. Half of the face was treated with fractional CO_2 laser and the other half with the same laser combined with bipolar radiofrequency.

We set the fractional laser with the following therapeutic protocol: Power: 15 W; Dwell time: 1 ms; Spacing: 500 μm; Stack: 1–3; Pulse mode: DP; Scanning mode: SmartTrack. The other half treated with the fractional laser + radiofrequency combination used the same protocol as above with the addition of RF with 25 W for 2.5 s.

Clinical pictures of the treated areas showed a gradual improvement in the skin structure and a reduction in the depth of the acne scars either on the side of the face treated with fractional laser combined with RF or on the side treated with only fractional laser.

However, the dermoscopic examination performed before and after each treatment has clearly shown a greater improvement in the scars treated with the fractional laser + RF compared to those treated with the fractional laser alone. These results were confirmed at 30 days follow-up in 8/10 (80%) treated patients. In all these cases, the dermoscopic examination has clearly demonstrated more positive results in the scars treated with the combined method of fractional RF than those treated with the fractional laser alone.

It is interesting to note, however, that the initial results obtained in the scars treated with the fractionated fractional laser-RF method were also confirmed at subsequent dermoscopic follow-ups, while in the short term the scars treated with the fractional laser alone did not show any significant improvement with dermoscopy, although they improved in subsequent follow-ups. These results probably show that the RF action stimulates the reabsorption of the fibrous component of the scar already after the first days of post-treatment, while the component stimulated by the fractional laser only involves a remodeling action of the dermis that is visible only from 45 to 60 days after treatment.

On the contrary, in post-trauma scars, the dermoscopic examination clearly showed that the combined fractionated laser-RF treatment is far more effective both in the short term and in the long term than that performed with the fractional laser alone (Figs. 10.1 and 10.2).

In the case of partially pigmented post-trauma scars, the combined use of fractional CO_2 laser and RF has shown excellent results both on the structure and on the accessory pigmentary component of the scar after a single session. These results can be further improved in subsequent sessions.

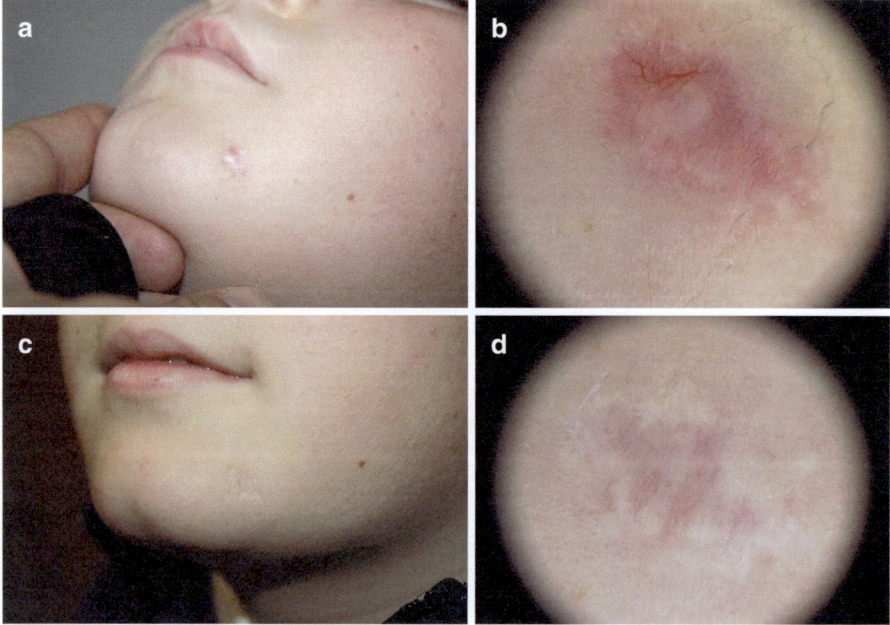

Fig. 10.1 (**a**) Clinical picture of a hypertrophic post-traumatic scar in a child before any treatment. (**b**) Dermoscopy image of the lesion. (**c**) Clinical image after three IPL sessions. (**d**) Dermoscopic exam highlights a complete clearance of the vessels' reticular and a change in the scar's color from red to white. (Courtesy of Dr. Domenico Piccolo, Skin Center Avezzano, Italy)

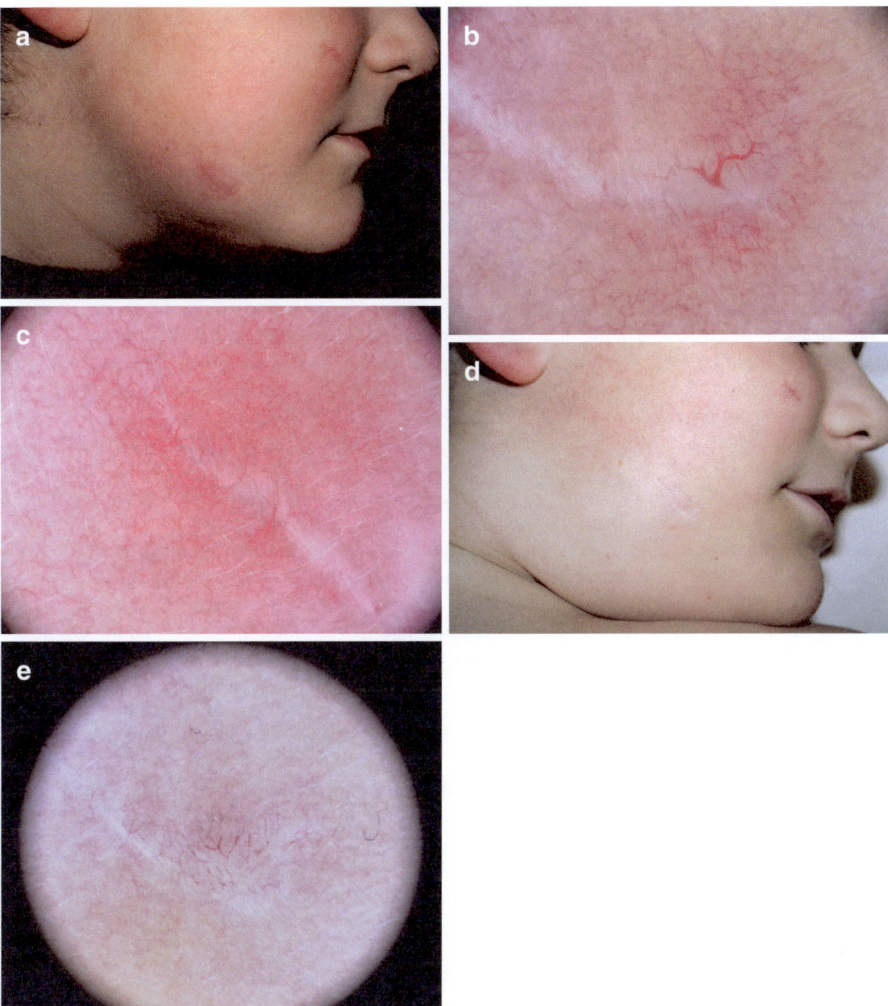

Fig. 10.2 (**a**) Clinical picture of a hypertrophic post-traumatic scar in a child before any treatment. (**b**) Dermoscopy image of the lesion revealing the neovascularization of the scar. (**c**) Dermoscopic image after one IPL session. (**d**) Clinical picture after two IPL sessions. (**e**) Dermoscopic exam highlights a complete clearance of the vessels' reticular and a change in the scar's color from red to white. (Courtesy of Dr. Domenico Piccolo, Skin Center Avezzano, Italy)

References

Alster TS, Tanzi EL, Lazarus M. The use of fractional laser photothermolysis for the treatment of atrophic scars. Dermatol Surg. 2007;33:295–9.

Bae-Harboe YS, Graber EM. Easy as PIE (postinflammatory erythema). J Clin Aesthet Dermatol. 2013;6:46–7.

Campolmi P, Bonan P, Cannarozzo G, et al. Efficacy and safety evaluation of an innovative CO2 laser/radiofrequency device in dermatology. J Eur Acad Dermatol Venereol. 2013;27:1481–90.

Cannarozzo G, Sannino M, Tamburi F, et al. Deep pulse fractional CO2 laser combined with a radiofrequency system: results of a case series. Photomed Laser Surg. 2014;32:409–12.

Chan NPY, Ho SGY, Yeung CK, et al. The use of non-ablative fractional resurfacing in Asian acne scar patients. Lasers Surg Med. 2010;42:870–5.

Chapas AM, Brightman L, Sukal S, et al. Successful treatment of acneiform scarring with CO 2 ablative fractional resurfacing. Lasers Surg Med. 2008;40:381–6.

Cho SB, Lee SJ, Cho S, et al. Non-ablative 1550-nm erbium-glass and ablative 10 600-nm carbon dioxide fractional lasers for acne scars: a randomized split-face study with blinded response evaluation. J Eur Acad Dermatol Venereol. 2010;24:921–5.

Clark E, Scerri L. Superficial and medium-depth chemical peels. J Clin Dermatol. 2008;26:209–18.

Connolly D, Vu HL, Mariwalla K, et al. Acne scarring-pathogenesis, evaluation, and treatment options. J Clin Aesthet Dermatol. 2017;10:12–23.

Cotterill JA, Cunliffe WJ. Suicide in dermatologic patients. Br J Dermatol. 1997;137:246–50.

Davis EC, Callender VD. Postinflammatory hyperpigmentation: a review of the epidemiology, clinical features, and treatment options in skin of color. J Clin Aesthet Dermatol. 2010;3:20–31.

Degitz K, Ochsendorf F. Acne. J Dtsch Dermatol Ges. 2017;15:709–22.

Degitz K, Placzek M, Borelli C, et al. Pathophysiology of acne. J Dtsch Dermatol Ges. 2007;5:316–23.

Dreno B, Khammari A, Orain N, et al. ECCA grading scale: an original validated acne scar grading scale for clinical practice in dermatology. Dermatology. 2007;214:46–51.

Elsaie ML, Ibrahim SM, Saudi W. Ablative fractional 10 600 nm carbon dioxide laser versus non-ablative fractional 1540 nm erbium-glass laser in Egyptian post-acne scar patients. J Lasers Med Sci. 2018;9:32–5.

Fabbrocini G, Annunziata MC, D'Arco V, et al. Acne Scars: Pathogenesis, Classification and Treatment. Dermatology Research and Practice. 2010;2010:893080.

Fearmonti R, Bond J, Erdmann D, et al. A review of scar scales and scar measuring devices. Eplasty. 2010;10:e43.

Fernandes M, Pinheiro NM, Crema VO, et al. Effects of microdermabrasion on skin rejuvenation. J Cosmet Laser Ther. 2014;16:26–31.

Fife D. Practical evaluation and management of atrophic acne scars: tips for the general dermatologist. J Clin Aesthet Dermatol. 2011;4:50–7.

Ghodsi SZ, Orawa H, Zouboulis CC. Prevalence, severity, and severity risk factors of acne in high school pupils: a community-based study. J Invest Dermatol. 2009;129:2136–41.

Gollnick HP. From new findings in acne pathogenesis to new approaches in treatment. J Eur Acad Dermatol Venereol. 2015;29(Suppl 5):1–7.

Gollnick HP, Zouboulis CC. Not all acne is acne vulgaris. Dtsch Arztebl Int. 2014;111:301–12.

Goodman G. Post acne scarring: a review. J Cosmet Laser Ther. 2003;5:77–95.

Goodman GJ, Baron JA. Postacne scarring: a qualitative global scarring grading system. Dermatol Surg. 2006;32:1458–66.

Gotkin RH, Sarnoff DS. A preliminary study on the safety and efficacy of a novel fractional CO_2 laser with synchronous radiofrequency delivery. J Drugs Dermatol. 2014;13:299–304.

Goulden V, Stables GI, Cunliffe WJ. Prevalence of facial acne in adults. J Am Acad Dermatol. 1999;41:577–80.

Gozali MV, Zhou B. Effective treatments of atrophic acne scars. J Clin Aesthet Dermatol. 2015;8:33–40.

Grevelink JM, White VR. Concurrent use of laser skin resurfacing and punch excision in the treatment of facial acne scarring. Dermatol Surg. 1998;24:527–30.

Hayashi N, Miyachi Y, Kawashima M. Prevalence of scars and "mini-scars", and their impact on quality of life in Japanese patients with acne. J Dermatol. 2015;42:690–6.

Hirsch RJ, Cohen JL. Soft tissue augmentation. Cutis. 2006;78:165–72.

Holland DB, Jeremy AH, Roberts SG, et al. Inflammation in acne scarring: a comparison of the responses in lesions from patients prone and not prone to scar. Br J Dermatol. 2004;150:72–81.

Jacob CI, Dover JS, Kaminer MS. Acne scarring: a classification system and review of treatment options. J Am Acad Dermatol. 2001;45:109–17.

James WD. Clinical practice. Acne. N Engl J Med. 2005;352:1463–72.

Kilkenny M, Merlin K, Plunkett A, et al. The prevalence of common skin conditions in Australian school students: 3. Acne vulgaris. Br J Dermatol. 1998;139:840–5.

Koo J. The psychosocial impact patients' perceptions. J Am Acad Dermatol. 1995;32(Suppl):S26–30.

Koo JY, Smith LL. Psychologic aspects of acne. Pediatr Dermatol. 1991;8:185–8.

Kraning KK, Odland GF. Morbidity and cost of dermatologic diseases. J Investig Dermatol. 1979;73:395–401.

Lauermann FT, Almeida HL Jr, Duquia RP, et al. Acne scars in 18-year-old male adolescents: a population-based study of prevalence and associated factors. An Bras Dermatol. 2016;91:291–5.

Layton AM. Optimal management of acne to prevent scarring and psychological sequelae. Am J Clin Dermatol. 2001;2:135–41.

Layton AM, Henderson CA, Cunliffe WJ. A clinical evaluation of acne scarring and its incidence. Clin Exp Dermatol. 1994;19:303–8.

Mahmoud BH, Srivastava D, Janiga JJ, et al. Safety and efficacy of erbium-doped yttrium aluminum garnet fractionated laser for treatment of acne scars in type IV to VI skin. Dermatol Surg. 2010;36:602–9.

Manstein D, Herron GS, Sink RK. Fractional photothermolysis: a new concept for cutaneous remodeling using microscopic patterns of thermal injury. Lasers Surg Med. 2004;34:426–38.

Manuskiatti W, Triwongwaranat D, Varothai S, et al. Efficacy and safety of a carbon- dioxide ablative fractional resurfacing device for treatment of atrophic acne scars in Asians. J Am Acad Dermatol. 2010;63:274–83.

Moradi Tuchayi S, Makrantonaki E, Ganceviciene R, et al. Acne vulgaris. Nat Rev Dis Primers. 2015;1:15029.

O'Daniel TG. Multimodal management of atrophic acne scarring in the aging face. Aesthet Plast Surg. 2011;35:1143–50.

Orentreich DS, Orentreich N. Subcutaneous incisionless (subcision) surgery for the correction of depressed scars and wrinkles. Dermatol Surg. 1995;21:543–9.

Pavlidis AI, Katsambas AD. Therapeutic approaches to reducing atrophic acne scarring. Clin Dermatol. 2017;35(2):190–4.

Poli F, Dreno B, Verschoore M. An epidemiological study of acne in female adults: results of a survey conducted in France. J Eur Acad Dermatol Venereol. 2001;15:541–5.

Reinholz M, Schwaiger H, Heppt MV, et al. Comparison of two kinds of lasers in the treatment of acne scars. Facial Plast Surg. 2015;31:523–31.

Saint-Jean M, Khammari A, Jasson F, et al. Different cutaneous innate immunity profiles in acne patients with and without atrophic scars. Eur J Dermatol. 2016;26:68–74.

Stratigos AJ, Katsambas AD. Optimal management of recalcitrant disorders of hyperpigmentation in dark-skinned patients. Am J Clin Dermatol. 2004;5(3):161–8.

Tan JK, Bhate K. A global perspective on the epidemiology of acne. Br J Dermatol. 2015;172(Suppl 1):3–12.

Tan J, Bourdès V, Bissonnette R, Petit B, Eng L, Reynier P, Khammari A, et al. Prospective study of pathogenesis of atrophic acne scars and role of macular erythema. J Drugs Dermatol. 2017a;16:566–72.

Tan J, Kang S, Leyden J. Prevalence and risk factors of acne scarring among patients consulting dermatologists in the USA. J Drugs Dermatol. 2017b;16:97–102.

Tenna S, Cogliandro A, Piombino L, et al. Combined use of fractional CO2 laser and radio-frequency waves to treat acne scars: a pilot study on 15 patients. J Cosmet Laser Ther. 2012;14:166–71.

Walgrave SE, Ortiz AE, MacFalls HT, Elkeeb L, Truitt AK, Tournas JA, et al. Evaluation of a novel fractional resurfacing device for treatment of acne scarring. Lasers Surg Med. 2009;41:122–7.

Yeung CK, Teo LH, Xiang LH, Chan HH. A community-based epidemiological study of acne vulgaris in Hong Kong adolescents. Acta Derm Venereol. 2002;82:104–7.

You HJ, Kim DW, Yoon ES, Park SH. Comparison of four different lasers for acne scars: resurfacing and fractional lasers. J Plast Reconstr Aesthet Surg. 2016;69:e87–95.

Dermoscopy Applied to Laser and IPL Treatments: Keloids and Hypertrophic Scars

11

Keloid is a term derived from the Greek word χηλή, chele, which means crab's claw, and describes the lateral growth of tissue into unaffected skin (Bayat et al. 2003). Both keloids and hypertrophic scars are lesions characterized by excessive proliferation of fibroblasts and collagen synthesis. By definition, keloids extend beyond the margins of the original skin wound while hypertrophic scars are limited to the area of injury (Murray 1994; Brissett and Sherris 2001). Both lesions may result from abnormal wound healing in response to a vast array of traumatic events including burns, surgery, piercing, skin lacerations, acne, insect bites, etc. Hypertrophic scars usually show a rapid growth phase for up to 6 months, and then gradually regress over a period of a few years, eventually leading to flat scars with no further symptoms (Gauglitz et al. 2011; Hunasgi et al. 2013). Keloids, in contrast, may develop up to several years after minor injuries, arising from a mature scar, or can occur as spontaneous lesions, and do not regress spontaneously (Burd and Huang 2005).

The worldwide prevalence of keloids varies according to ethnicity. Although keloids can appear in individuals of all ethnic backgrounds, except albinos, they are most commonly seen in individuals of African, Asian, and Hispanic and Mediterranean descent. Dark-skinned individuals are at an increased risk of 15–20 times to form keloids than their lighter-skinned counterparts (Brissett and Sherris 2001). It has been estimated that the incidence of keloid formation in both black and Hispanic population is as high as 16%, with higher frequencies during puberty and pregnancy (Chike-Obi et al. 2009). In addition, the occurrence of keloids and hypertrophic scars has equal sex distribution and can occur at every age, even though its prevalence is higher between the ages of 10 and 30 (Ramakrishnan et al. 1974).

Although most keloids occur sporadically, familial keloid cases have also been reported, reflecting the importance of genetic factors among these families (Marneros et al. 2001; Omo-Dare 1975). The pattern of inheritance observed in these families is consistent with an autosomal dominant model with incomplete

---

The contents of this book are partially based on the Italian language edition: "*The Usefulness of Dermoscopy in Laser and IPL Treatments*", Domenico Piccolo, © DEKA M.E.L.A Srl 2012.

clinical penetrance and variable expression (Shih and Bayat 2010). Several genes have been implicated in the etiology of keloids, but to date no single mutation of a gene has been recognized as responsible.

Clinically, the keloids appear as protruding fixed, irregular, slightly tender nodules, with well-circumscribed margins, a shiny surface, and sometimes telangiectasia. The color is pink to purple and can be accompanied by hyperpigmentation. In contrast, the hypertrophic scar has a similar appearance, but is commonly linear following the shape of the wound. Both lesions are generally itchy, but keloids can even be the source of significant pain and hyperesthesia (Niessen et al. 1999). Keloids can often be quite disfiguring, expanding far beyond the initiation site and embracing entire anatomical areas. When a keloid occurs near a flexor or extensor area, the patient may experience reduced limb mobility. Hypertrophic scars occur more frequently on the shoulders, neck, presternum, knees, and ankles, while keloids are often seen on the anterior chest, upper arms, cheeks, and ear lobes. However, the back side of the ear lobe is the most frequently involved site. Unusual positions for these growths include eyelids, genitals, palms, and soles (Robles and Berg 2007). Furthermore, keloids have a greater tendency to recur after excision (45–100%), while the new formation of hypertrophic scars is rare after its excision (10%) (Verhaegen et al. 2009).

The diagnosis of keloids or hypertrophic scars is based on the clinical aspect and on the history of a previous trauma or surgery. Biopsy is justified only in case of borderline lesions and lesions that mimic atypical infections or neoplasms (Ogawa et al. 2009).

Until now, the exact pathophysiology of keloids and hypertrophic scars remains poorly understood and the possible underlying cause is largely elusive (Alster and Tanzi 2003). The alterations of cellular signals that control proliferation and inflammation, in particular cytokine overexpression and growth factors, may be related to the disordered and increased production of collagen by fibroblasts and to the new dense growth of blood vessels, typically observed in keloid and hypertrophic scars (Al-Attar et al. 2006; Dong et al. 2013).

Understanding the pathophysiology of these lesions is critical to advancing the field and to developing optimal preventive and treatment strategies. Keloids often have a functional, cosmetic, or psychological impact on patients (Bock et al. 2006); therefore, there is a strong need for an effective and safe treatment.

Nowadays, the management of keloids and hypertrophic scars remains a challenge, mainly due to the complex pathophysiological mechanism, the lack of adequate model systems to evaluate the therapeutic efficacy, the difficulties in quantifying the changes in the appearance of the scar and of the limited amount of data derived from well-designed perspectives, and randomized controlled clinical trials (Gold et al. 2014). There is no single therapeutic method suitable for all types of scars (Leventhal et al. 2006).

The therapeutic approach is selected based on the type of injury (position, depth, size), patient's age, past response to treatment, aesthetic outcome, patient's willingness to undergo topical or invasive therapy, as well as the patient's economic conditions (Gupta and Sharma 2011).

It is important to note that it is difficult to eradicate keloids, and some of the modalities may be associated with adverse effects and high recurrence rates (Mamalis et al. 2014; Jackson et al. 2001). Therefore, to date, it remains much more efficient to prevent excessive scarring than to treat it. Given the complexity of the wound healing process, a multidisciplinary approach to the management of these injuries is widely recommended. Combination therapy has been shown to be more effective than monotherapy.

11.1   Treatment Options

Topical treatments include silicone gels and sheeting (Berman et al. 2007; Mustoe 2008), pressure dressings and pressure earrings (Leung and Ng 1980), aggressive deep-tissue massage as well as imiquimod 5% cream (Berman et al. 2009). Invasive treatments include intralesional injections of triamcinolone (Lee et al. 2001), bleomycin (Saray and Güleç 2005; Naeini et al. 2006), verapamil (D'Andrea et al. 2002) and 5-fluorouracil (5-FU) (Davison et al. 2009), cryosurgery (Zouboulis et al. 1993; Har-Shai et al. 2008), surgical excision (Kim et al. 2005; Lee et al. 2001), and radiation (Ogawa et al. 2007).

Other methods used to treat these lesions are laser and light-based therapies that can be grouped into the following three categories (Mamalis et al. 2014): ablative lasers, nonablative lasers and noncoherent light sources. It is worth noting that different lasers have different effects on scars.

Ablative lasers include the 2940-nm erbium-doped:yttrium, aluminum, and garnet (Er:YAG) laser and the 10,600-nm carbon dioxide (CO_2). They use water as a target chromophore in skin, and therefore they can provoke local tissue destruction.

Nonablative lasers include pulsed dye laser (PDL), the 1064-nm neodymium-doped:yttrium, aluminum, and garnet (Nd:YAG) laser, and the 532-nm neodymium-doped:vanadate (Nd:Van) laser. Through selective photothermolysis, PDL targets hemoglobin chromophore and coagulates the capillaries sited within the reticular dermis, thus resulting in the destruction of pathologic neo-angiogenesis (de las Alas et al. 2012). This leads to hypoxemia which in turn may alter the local collagen production or may deprive a scar of nutrients to prevent scar hypertrophy (Paquet et al. 2001). In addition to its vascular specificity, PDL may produce a direct effect on collagen and cause keloid fibroblast functional modification. In particular, PDL can directly suppress the production of fibroblast collagen since the overheating of collagen can cause the dissolution of disulfide bonds and the consequent realignment of collagen fibers with a reduced proliferation of fibroblasts (Abergel et al. 1984). Furthermore, a decrease in mast cells observed after treatment suggested that PDL presumably produces an indirect effect, since the histamine released by mast cells is able to improve collagen synthesis.

Noncoherent light sources include intense pulsed light therapy (IPL), light-emitting diode phototherapy (LED), and photodynamic therapy (PDT). The basic IPL mechanism is not fully understood, yet. Given that it affects both melanin and vascular structure, IPL most likely acts on vascular proliferation, which is essential for the overgrowth of collagen, as well as on the pigmentation resulting from scar formation, thus improving the appearance and/or symptoms of hypertrophic scars and keloids (Kontoes et al. 2003; Piccolo et al. 2014). The best results after several IPL treatments are more evident after a few months. This is probably due to the inhibition of the vascular action caused by the IPL on the scar tissue and to the subsequent proliferation of the neocollagen. LED phototherapy can treat these lesions by photomodulating the mitochondrial cytochrome C oxidase and thereby altering intracellular signaling (Huang et al. 2011). Finally, PDT may be another therapeutic option as it causes the generation of free radicals of reactive oxygen species (with a cytotoxic effect), alterations in the synthesis and degradation of the extracellular matrix, and modulates the expression of cytokines and growth factors (Nie 2011).

Among the lasers mentioned above, today, PDL (585–595 nm) has become the standard of care for keloid and hypertrophic scars. In fact, various studies have shown that PDL can induce a significant overall clinical improvement in terms of vascularization, height, consistency, color, and flexibility of scars (Lupton and Alster 2002; Bouzari et al. 2007) and can resolve scar-related symptoms such as the itch. Aslter et al. reported an improvement in all the factors listed above ranging from 57% to 83%, after one or two PDL treatments, respectively (Alster 1994). However, efficacy in thick keloids or thick hypertrophic scars (>1 cm) may be limited since the PDL has an approximate penetration depth of 1.2 mm. In these cases, PDL therapy combined with intralesional corticosteroids or injections of 5-fluorouracil or other lasers such as the fractionated CO_2 laser has been shown to improve clinical outcomes (Khatri et al. 2011). Purpura is the main side effect of PDL, especially when using PDL at 585 nm.

A good alternative to PDL with similar results in the clinical improvement of scars and a lower risk of purpura is IPL. Most clinicians prefer IPL because it is less invasive, requires fewer therapeutic sessions to achieve desirable results, is more flexible, and can be used in different therapeutic skin purposes (Ross 2006). Bellew et al. (2005) have shown that IPL is as effective as 595 nm PDL with greater, however, improvement in textural smoothing components of scars. Kontoes et al. (2003) reported an improvement of over 75% in the pigmentation of hypertrophic scars, an improvement of more than 50% in asphalt scars, and a 50% reduction in the size and thickness of hypertrophic scars. These data were further confirmed in a retrospective study that assessed the efficacy and safety of IPL in the scar treatment of 109 patients, suggesting that IPL is effective not only in improving the appearance of hypertrophic scars and keloids, but also in reducing the height, redness, and hardness of the scars (Erol et al. 2008).

11.2   The Validity of Dermoscopy in the Treatment of Keloids and Hypertrophic Scars

The use of dermoscopy has proved very effective in the treatment of keloids and hypertrophic scars. Before the treatment (Figs. 11.1a, b and 11.2a, b) the dermoscopic examination shows the presence of possible pigmentation and

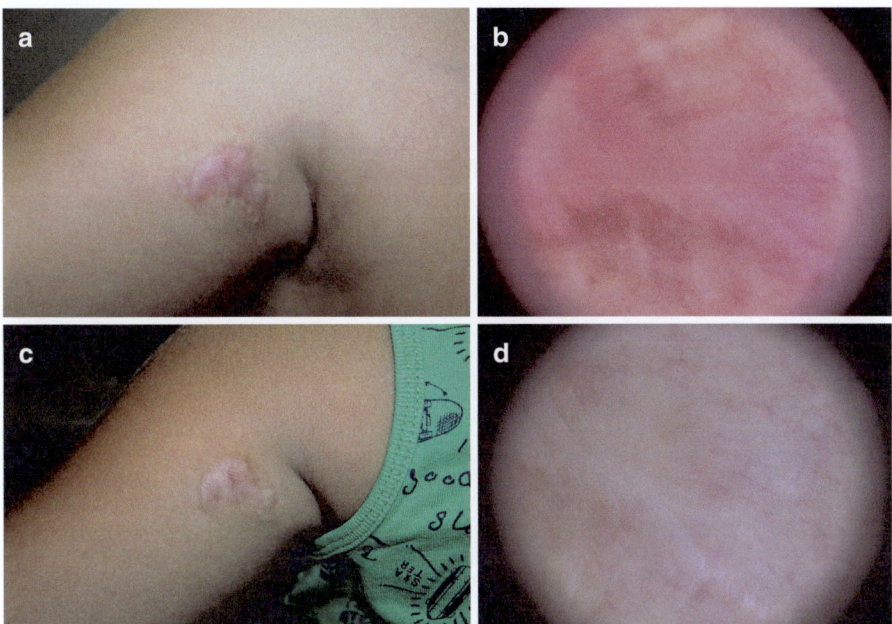

Fig. 11.1 (**a**) Clinical picture of a keloid on the right arm of a child before any treatment. (**b**) Dermoscopy image of the lesion. (**c**) Clinical image after three IPL sessions. (**d**) Dermoscopic exam highlights a complete clearance of the vessels' reticular and a change in the scar's color from red to white. (Courtesy of Dr. Domenico Piccolo, Skin Center Avezzano, Italy)

neo-angiogenesis responsible for cicatricial hypertrophy. The simultaneous presence of two different chromophores (melanin and hemoglobin) demonstrates that dermoscopy also helps the therapeutic choice by identifying the targets to be struck with maximum precision. Immediately after treatment with IPL dermoscopy (Figs. 11.1c and 11.2c) the color change of the vascularized part of the lesion is highlighted from blue to red. After three treatments with IPL, the dermoscopic examination shows how the pigmentary component of the scar and the residual vascularization have completely disappeared. Five treatment sessions with IPL dermoscopy show the complete disappearance of the components (pigmentary and vascular) with excellent clinical results (Figs. 11.1d and 11.2d).

Same results have been obtained in a young boy with a keloid of the right arm, treated with both fractional CO_2 laser and dye laser.

In the case of hypertrophic scars resulting from thyroidectomies, dermoscopy helps to identify the newly formed vessels responsible for the problem (Fig. 11.3a, b), thus allowing the selection of the most suitable treatment (dye laser or IPL) to strike these vessels with maximum precision. The purpose of this treatment is to eliminate the neo-angiogenesis and therefore obtain a smoothing effect from the scar. Dermoscopy performed at the end of the treatment shows the disappearance of the treated vessels (Fig. 11.3c, d).

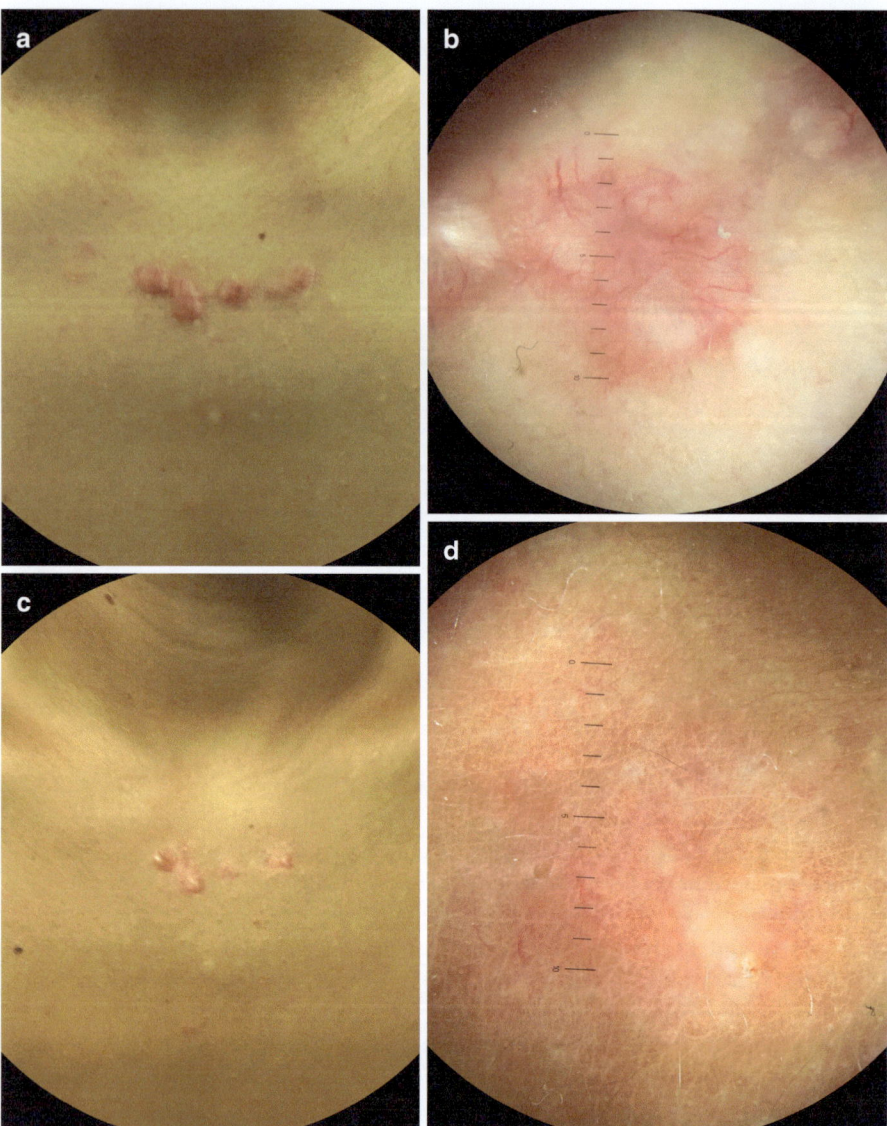

Fig. 11.2 (**a**) Clinical picture of a keloid on a post-traumatic scar on the décolleté of a young woman before any treatment. (**b**) Dermoscopy image of the lesion highlighting the neoangiogenesis of the scar. (**c**) Clinical image after two IPL sessions. (**d**) Dermoscopic exam highlights a complete clearance of the neoangiogenesis at the end of the treatment. (Courtesy of Dr. Domenico Piccolo, Skin Center Avezzano, Italy)

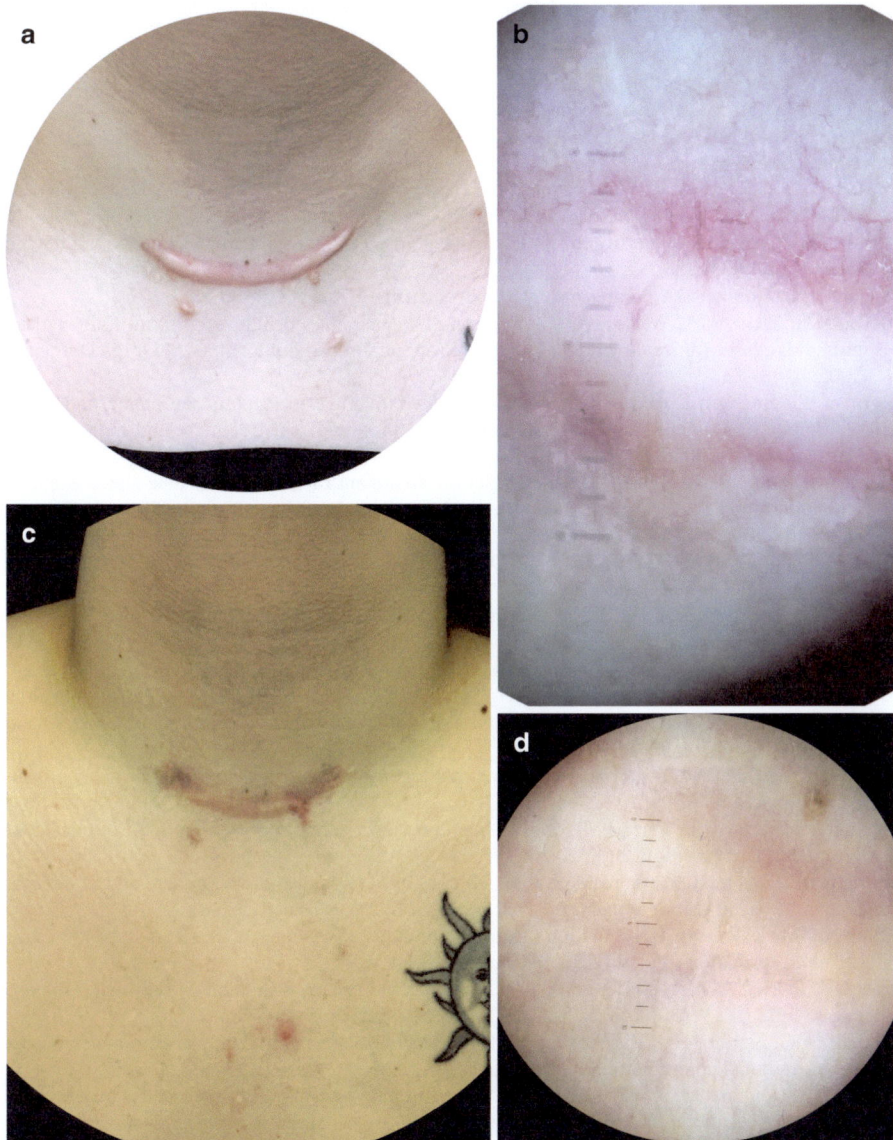

Fig. 11.3 (**a**) Clinical picture of a keloid after a thyroidectomy in a young woman before any treatment. (**b**) Dermoscopy image of the lesion highlighting the neoangiogenesis of the scar. (**c**) Clinical image after two IPL sessions. (**d**) Dermoscopic exam highlights a complete disappearance of the neoangiogenesis at the end of the treatment. (Courtesy of Dr. Domenico Piccolo, Skin Center Avezzano, Italy)

References

Abergel RP, Meeker CA, Lam TS, et al. Control of connective tissue metabolism by lasers: recent developments and future prospects. J Am Acad Dermatol. 1984;11:1142–50.

Al-Attar A, Mess S, Thomassen JM, et al. Keloid pathogenesis and treatment. Plast Reconstr Surg. 2006;117:286–300.

Alster TS. Improvement of erythematous and hypertrophic scars by the 585-nm flashlamp- pumped pulsed dye laser. Ann Plast Surg. 1994;32:186–90.

Alster TS, Tanzi EL. Hypertrophic scars and keloids: etiology and management. Am J Clin Dermatol. 2003;4:235.

Bayat A, McGrouther DA, Ferguson MWJ. Skin scarring. BMJ. 2003;326:88.

Bellew SG, Weiss MA, Weiss RA. Comparison of intense pulsed light to 595-nm long- pulsed pulsed dye laser for treatment of hypertrophic surgical scars: a pilot study. J Drugs Dermatol. 2005;4:448–52.

Berman B, Perez OA, Konda S, et al. A review of the biologic effects, clinical efficacy, and safety of silicone elastomer sheeting for hypertrophic and keloid scar treatment and management. Dermatol Surg. 2007;33:1291–303.

Berman B, Harrison-Balestra C, Perez OA, et al. Treatment of keloid scars post-shave excision with imiquimod 5% cream: a prospective, double-blind, placebo-controlled pilot study. J Drugs Dermatol. 2009;8:455.

Bock O, Schmid-Ott G, Malewski P, et al. Quality of life of patients with keloid and hypertrophic scarring. Arch Dermatol Res. 2006;297:433–8.

Bouzari N, Davis SC, Nouri K. Laser treatment of keloids and hypertrophic scars. Int J Dermatol. 2007;46:80–8.

Brissett AE, Sherris DA. Scar contractures, hypertrophic scars, and keloids. Facial Plast Surg. 2001;17:263–72.

Burd A, Huang L. Hypertrophic response and keloid diathesis: two very different forms of scar. Plast Reconstr Surg. 2005;116:150e–7e.

Chike-Obi C, Cole PD, Brissett AE. Keloids: pathogenesis, clinical features, and management. Semin Plast Surg. 2009;23:178–84.

D'Andrea F, Brongo S, Ferraro G, et al. Prevention and treatment of keloids with intralesional verapamil. Dermatology. 2002;204:60–2.

Davison SP, Dayan JH, Clemens MW, et al. Efficacy of intralesional 5-fluorouracil and triamcinolone in the treatment of keloids. Aesthet Surg J. 2009;29:40–6.

Dong X, Mao S, Wen H. Upregulation of proinflammatory genes in skin lesions may be the cause of keloid formation (review). Biomed Rep. 2013;1:833–6.

Erol OO, Gurlek A, Agaoglu G, et al. Treatment of hypertrophic scars and keloids using intense pulsed light (IPL). Aesthet Plast Surg. 2008;32:902–9.

Gauglitz GG, Korting HC, Pavicic T, et al. Hypertrophic scarring and keloids: pathomechanisms and current and emerging treatment strategies. Mol Med. 2011;17:113–25.

Gold MH, McGuire M, Mustoe TA, et al. International Advisory Panel on Scar Management. Updated international clinical recommendations on scar management: part 2--algorithms for scar prevention and treatment. Dermatol Surg. 2014;40:825–31.

Gupta S, Sharma VK. Standard guidelines of care: keloids and hypertrophic scars. Indian J Dermatol Venereol Leprol. 2011;77:94–100.

Har-Shai Y, Brown W, Labbéé D, et al. Intralesional cryosurgery for the treatment of hypertrophic scars and keloids following aesthetic surgery: the results of a prospective observational study. Int J Low Extrem Wounds. 2008;7:169–75.

Huang YY, Sharma SK, Carroll J, et al. Biphasic dose response in low level light therapy - an update. Dose Response. 2011;9:602–18.

Hunasgi S, Koneru A, Vanishree M, et al. A case report and review of pathophysiology and differences between keloid and hypertrophic scars. J Oral Maxillofac Pathol. 2013;17:116–20.

Jackson IT, Bhageshpur R, DiNick V, et al. Investigation of recurrence rates among earlobe keloids utilizing various postoperative therapeutic modalities. Eur J Plast Surg. 2001;24:88–95.

Khatri KA, Mahoney DL, McCartney MJ. Laser scar revision: a review. J Cosmet Laser Ther. 2011;13:54–62.

Kim DY, Kim ES, Eo SR, et al. A surgical approach for earlobe keloid: keloid fillet flap. Arch Facial Plast Surg. 2005;7:172–5.

Kontoes PP, Marayiannis KV, Vlachos SP. The use of intense pulsed light in the treatment of scars. Eur J Plast Surg. 2003;25:374–7.

de las Alas JM, Siripunvarapon AH, Dofitas BL. Pulsed dye laser for the treatment of keloid and hypertrophic scars: a systematic review. Expert Rev Med Devices. 2012;9:641–50.

Lee Y, Minn KW, Baek RM, et al. A new surgical treatment of keloid: keloid core excision. Ann Plast Surg. 2001;46:135–40.

Leung P, Ng M. Pressure treatment for hypertrophic scars resulting from burns. Burns. 1980;6:244.

Leventhal D, Furr M, Reiter D. Treatment of keloids and hypertrophic scars. Arch Facial Plast Surg. 2006;8:362–8.

Lupton JR, Alster TS. Laser scar revision. Dermatol Clin. 2002;20:55–65.

Mamalis AD, Lev-Tov H, Nguyen DH, et al. Laser and light-based treatment of Keloids--a review. J Eur Acad Dermatol Venereol. 2014;28:689–99.

Marneros AG, Norris JE, Olsen BR, et al. Clinical genetics of familial keloids. Arch Dermatol. 2001;137:1429–34.

Murray JC. Keloids and hypertrophic scars. Clin Dermatol. 1994;12:27–37.

Mustoe TA. Evolution of silicone therapy and mechanism of action in scar management. Aesthet Plast Surg. 2008;32:82–92.

Naeini FF, Najafian J, Ahmadpour K. Bleomycin tattooing as a promising therapeutic modality in large keloids and hypertrophic scars. Dermatol Surg. 2006;32:1023–9.

Nie Z. Is photodynamic therapy a solution for keloid? G Ital Dermatol Venereol. 2011;146:463–72.

Niessen F, Spauwen P, Schalkwijk J, et al. On the nature of hypertrophic scars and keloids: a review. Plast Reconstr Surg. 1999;104:1435–58.

Ogawa R, Miyashita T, Hyakusoku H, et al. Postoperative radiation protocol for keloids and hypertrophic scars: statistical analysis of 370 sites followed for over 18 months. Ann Plast Surg. 2007;59:688–91.

Ogawa R, Akaishi S, Hyakusoku H. Differential and exclusive diagnosis of diseases that resemble keloids and hypertrophic scars. Ann Plast Surg. 2009;62:660–4.

Omo-Dare P. Genetic studies on keloid. J Natl Med Assoc. 1975;67:428–32.

Paquet P, Hermanns JF, Piérard GE. Effect of the 585 nm flashlamp-pumped pulsed dye laser for the treatment of keloids. Dermatol Surg. 2001;27:171–4.

Piccolo D, Di Marcantonio D, Crisman G, et al. Unconventional use of intense pulsed light. Biomed Res Int. 2014;2014:618206.

Ramakrishnan KM, Thomas KP, Sundararajan CR. Study of 1,000 patients with keloids in South India. Plast Reconstr Surg. 1974;53:276–80.

Robles DT, Berg D. Abnormal wound healing: keloids. Clin Dermatol. 2007;25:26–32.

Ross EV. Laser versus intense pulsed light: competing technologies in dermatology. Lasers Surg Med. 2006;38:261–72.

Saray Y, Güleç AT. Treatment of keloids and hypertrophic scars with dermojet injections of bleomycin: a preliminary study. Int J Dermatol. 2005;44:777–84.

Shih B, Bayat A. Genetics of keloid scarring. Arch Dermatol Res. 2010;302:319–39.

Verhaegen PD, van Zuijlen PP, Pennings NM, et al. Differences in collagen architecture between keloid, hypertrophic scar, normotrophic scar, and normal skin: an objective histopathological analysis. Wound Repair Regen. 2009;17:649–56.

Zouboulis CC, Blume U, Büttner P, et al. Outcomes of cryosurgery in keloids and hypertrophic scars. A prospective consecutive trial of case series. Arch Dermatol. 1993;129:1146–51.

Dermoscopy Applied to Laser Treatments: Tattoos Removal

12

The term *tattoo* comes from the Polynesian word *tatau*, and it refers to an ornamental technique through the painting of the body. Since its origin, the tattooing technique envisaged that the decoration should last forever, but recently new techniques have been invented to give life to temporary tattoos, which disappear as the skin is washed (henna tattoos).

Currently, millions of people around the world show tattoos located almost everywhere in their bodies and, according to Kierstein L. and Kjelskau KC (2015), females have increased their interest in the world of tattoos and it can be estimated that 15% of women are tattooed compared to 13% of men.

There are many reasons to get tattooed, because a tattoo can represent both the search for individuality and belonging to a group (sports, social, ethnic, religious), but they may also communicate the most aesthetic sense of art or need to follow the fashion of the moment. Every individual has his/her reasons for getting a tattoo and so two people can choose the same symbol or design and have totally different reasons why they want to get that tattoo (Antoszewski et al. 2010; Carmen et al. 2012; Dickson et al. 2015).

Based on current literature two levels of medical risk and complications are associated with tattooing: mild and advanced. Mild complaints are referred to acute aseptic inflammatory reaction, inherent to tattoo placement or removal, followed by a wound healing process, while advanced complaints are more serious adverse reactions in tattoos, associated with objective symptoms and significant discomfort, requiring medical advice (Rahimi et al. 2018).

Although a systematic categorization of tattoo adverse events remains extremely challenging, tattoo reactions are more often subdivided in three main categories: (1) inflammatory including allergic contact dermatitis, photodermatitis, granulomatous and lichenoid reactions, and skin diseases localized on tattooed area (eczema, psoriasis, lichen, and morphea); (2) infections including bacterial, viral, or mycotic infections which can appear as superficial or with deep skin involvement; (3)

The contents of this book are partially based on the Italian language edition: "*The Usefulness of Dermoscopy in Laser and IPL Treatments*", Domenico Piccolo, © DEKA M.E.L.A Srl 2012.

neoplastic including keratoacanthoma, squamous cell and basal cell carcinoma, leiomyosarcoma, and melanoma (Bassi et al. 2014). The most frequent tattoo reactions concern allergic contact dermatitis, due to delayed hypersensitivity reaction to different pigments contained in the tattoos especially red ink, but also to chromium in green ink, cadmium in yellow ink, and cobalt in blue ink (Kaur et al. 2009; Glassy et al. 2012; Grimm and Cronin 2014). Complications associated with tattoo removal include hyper- and hypopigmentation, texture changes like scaring, local allergic responses to many tattoo pigments as well as ink retention despite multiple sessions.

At the same time, many patients came and requested a tattoo removal, both for aesthetic and psychological reasons. In our society (Italy), tattoos can represent a serious obstacle for the career, in particular for tattoos located on a visible part of the body.

12.1 Treatment Options

According to the literature, many methods of tattoo removal have been explored: dermabrasion, salabrasion, surgical excision, freeze-burning with liquid nitrogen, and, lately, lasers.

The most commonly used lasers for removing tattoos are the so-called Quality-Switched 1064-nm Nd:YAG. Because of its longer wavelength, higher fluency, and shorter pulse, it represents the gold standard treatment for black or dark blue/black tattoos. The use of lasers to remove tattoos was an important advance in dermatology. Quality-switched lasers emit short pulses of light (nanoseconds) to fragment pigments through selective photothermolysis. Up to now, they are considered the gold standard for tattoo removal. If performed in tanned skins or with the use of lasers with wavelengths of 532 or 694 nm, hypopigmentation may represent a side effect, probably due to the destruction of melanin in the basal layer of the epidermis, even though it is usually transient and repigmentation can occur spontaneously over time. However, achromic areas (as for vitiligo) can improve with sun exposure or phototherapy.

The use of high-energy lasers in intensely pigmented areas or by multiple laser treatments in the same area may result in achromatic scar, and it may be difficult to make a clinical distinction between achromic patches and achromic scars. Achromic scars can appear after the first laser sessions or develop only after the complete removal of the tattoo pigment. As with any scar, these lesions are difficult to treat because they do not repigment over time or with phototherapy. Moreover, since these scars are very superficial, intralesional infiltration is technically difficult.

In 2004, Fulton et al. (2004) reported the successful repigmentation of hypochromic scars using a multistep technique to remove areas of hypopigmentation associated with dermal fibrosis. This led us to search for a simpler and less invasive method to remove this type of fibrosis. A few months ago, Arbache et al. (2019) recently described a microinfusion drug delivery technique that uses needling and a tattoo machine using MMP® ("Microinfusão de Medicamentos na Pele," Portuguese acronym for "Microinfusion of Drugs in the Skin"). Tattoos are undeniable proof that this is an effective method to "inject" chemical substances into the dermis. MMP® has been successfully used to repigment idiopathic guttate hypomelanosis.

In 2009, Kirby W. et al. proposed the so-called Kirby–Desai Scale, based on six tattoo criteria (namely, skin phototype, location, tattoos' color, amount of ink, scarring, and layering), in the aim to offer a useful index to correlate with the number of treatment sessions required for satisfactory tattoo removal (Kirby et al. 2009).

In our experience with the "Q-Switched" 1064-nm Nd:YAG laser, some tattoos hesitate with some ghost effect, so that the tattoo is no more defined but still visible to the naked eye (Fig. 12.1a, b).

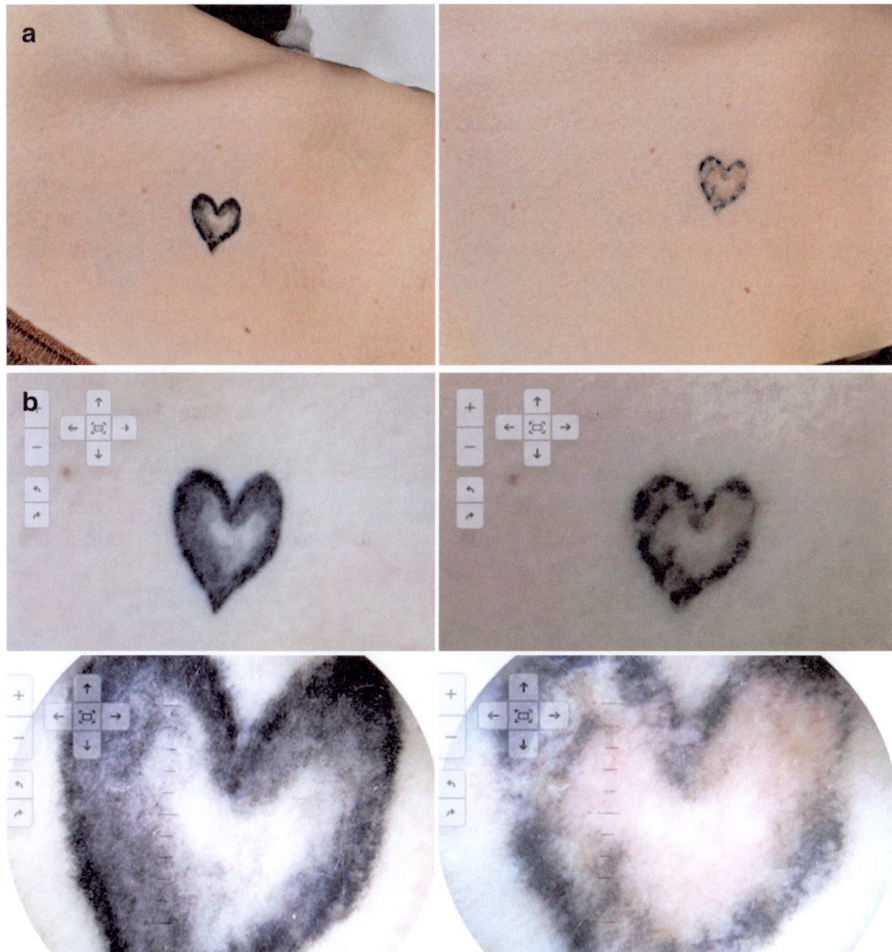

Fig. 12.1   (**a**) A tattoo before and after 40 days from the treatment. (**b**) Dermoscopic exam underlines a partial success of the treatment even though the tattoo is still clearly visible. (Courtesy of Dr. Domenico Piccolo, Skin Center Avezzano, Italy)

12.2   The Validity of Dermoscopy in Tattoos Removal

When a patient decides to remove a tattoo, one of the first questions asked to his/her dermatologist is how many sessions are needed, especially if they have a forthcoming military check up or job interview.

It is usually difficult to predict the exact number of sessions required because so many parameters can influence the result: size of tattoo, location in the body, tattoos' colors (black and dark blue are easier to remove than green and red), amount of ink, so the correct answer is that it will take a long time.

The clinical results obtained after the first sessions are not always so obvious, leading the patient to feel distrust and disappointment. The dermoscopic examination comes into play here, as it is able to highlight the differences in the color change of the tattoo not visible to the naked eye, thus demonstrating the effectiveness of the treatment, and in the majority of cases, dermoscopic images are accepted by the military investigating commission as proof of the treatment in progress (Figs. 12.2a–c, 12.3, 12.4, 12.5, 12.6a, b, and 12.7a–i). This is particularly important for colored tattoo, since black pigment is easier to treat, while red, yellow, and blue pigment are more resistant to QS treatment (Figs. 12.8a–i and 12.9a–q).

At the end of the treatment, some patients still notice the presence of the pigment in the treated area (Figs. 12.5, 12.6c, d, and 12.7j, k). In many cases, this was the result of the ghost effect, while in others the pigment could have been due to residual inflammation. This latter case is clearly detected by dermoscopy exam and by the software's filters (a pigmentary filter and a vascular filter are useful tools to examine the residual lesions in order to study the residual of pigments and the inflammatory response) (Figs. 12.6c, d and 12.7l, m), which makes it possible to avoid any additional treatments that would only increase inflammation and the risk of scarring.

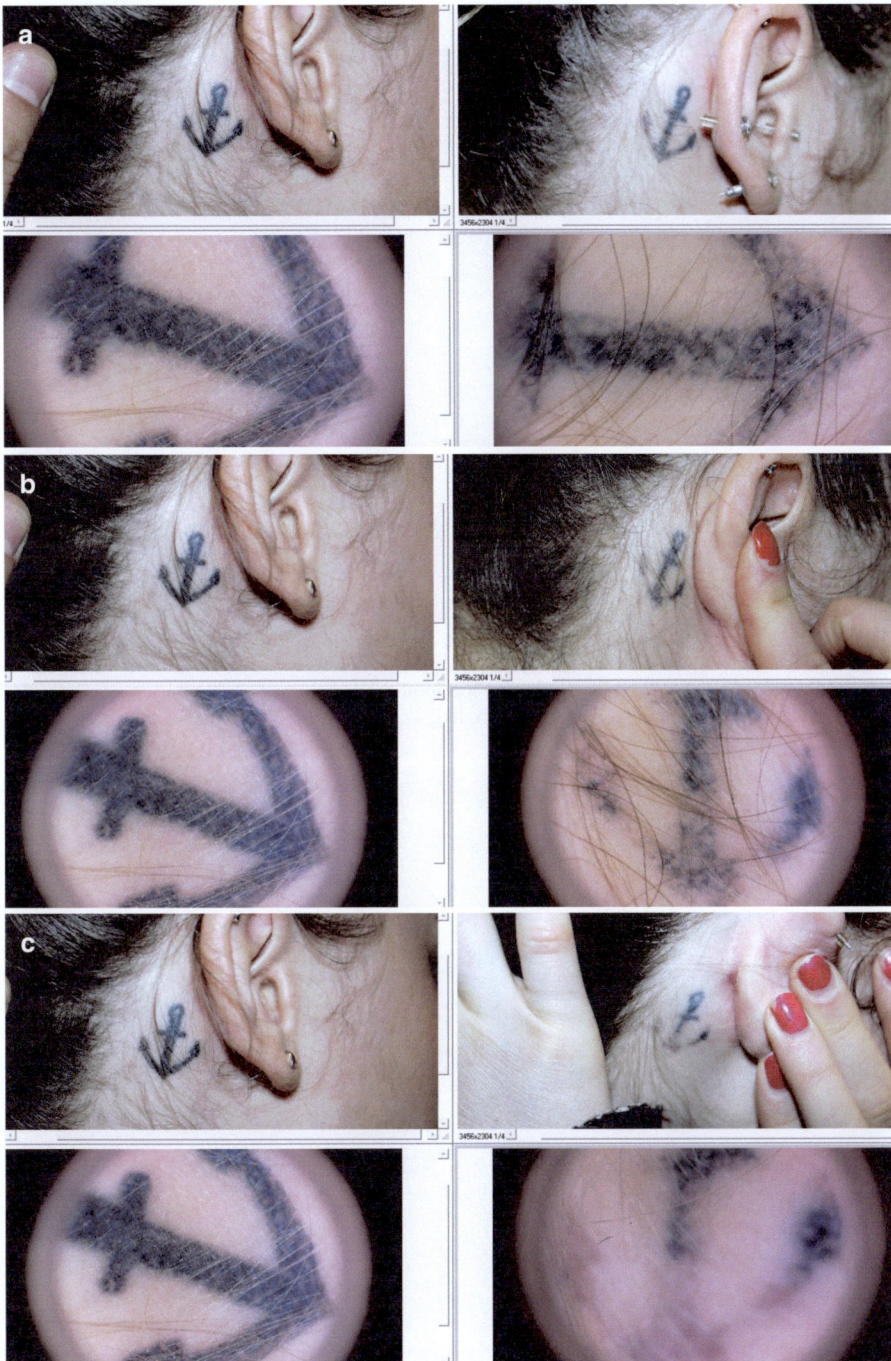

Fig. 12.2 (**a**) A tattoo before and after 1QS session (clinical and dermoscopic picture). (**b**) A tattoo before and after 2QS sessions (clinical and dermoscopic picture). (**c**) A tattoo before and after 3QS sessions (clinical and dermoscopic picture). (Courtesy of Dr. Domenico Piccolo, Skin Center Avezzano, Italy)

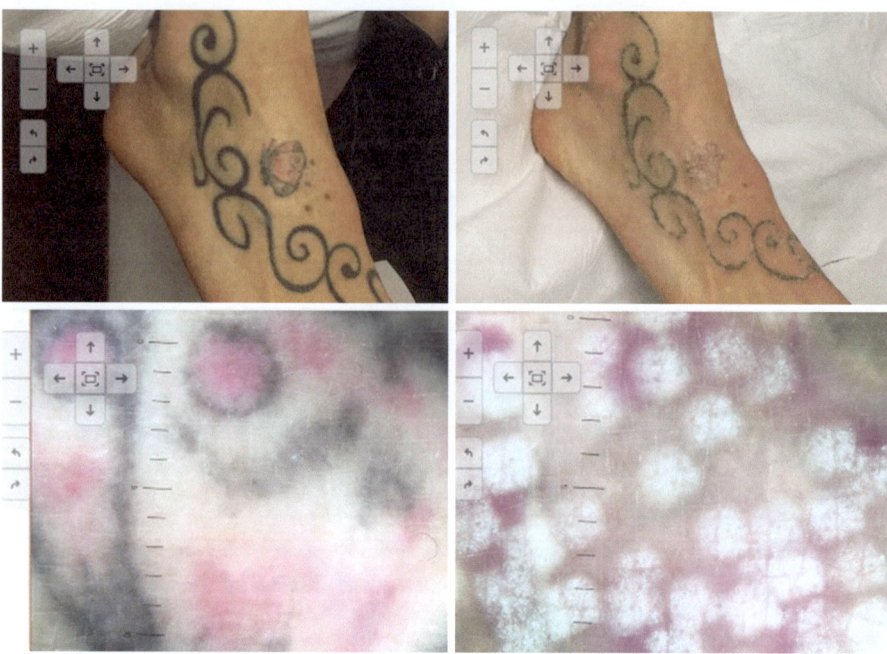

Fig. 12.3 A tattoo before and after 1QS session (clinical and dermoscopic picture). (Courtesy of Dr. Domenico Piccolo, Skin Center Avezzano, Italy)

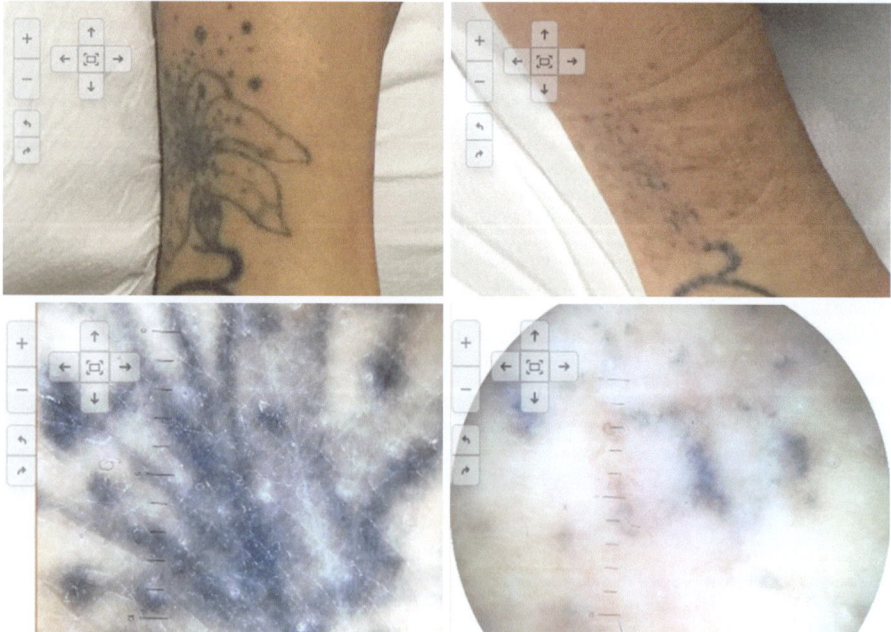

Fig. 12.4 A tattoo before and after 1QS session (clinical and dermoscopic picture). (Courtesy of Dr. Domenico Piccolo, Skin Center Avezzano, Italy)

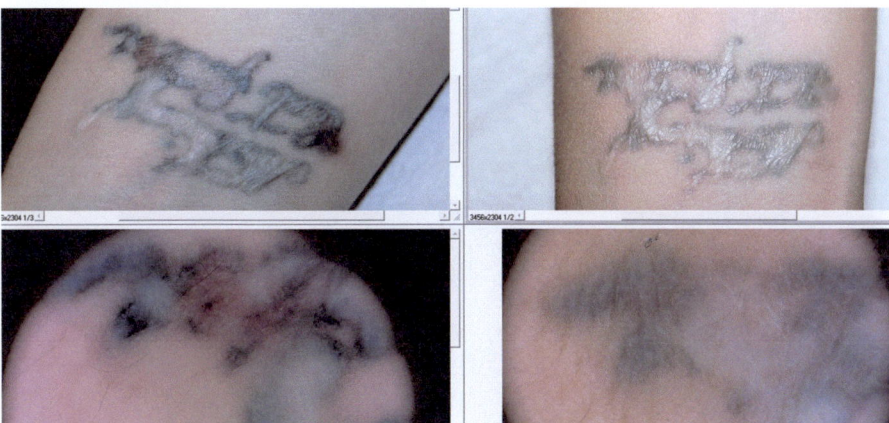

Fig. 12.5 A tattoo before and after 3QS sessions (clinical and dermoscopic picture). Please note the persistence of the pigment, highlighted by dermoscopic exam. (Courtesy of Dr. Domenico Piccolo, Skin Center Avezzano, Italy)

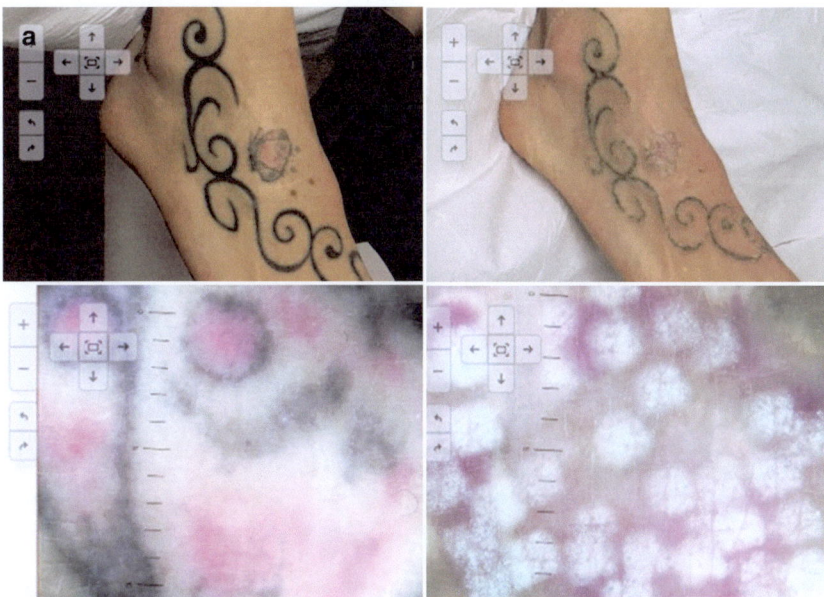

Fig. 12.6 (**a**) A tattoo before and immediately after 1QS session (clinical and dermoscopic picture). (**b**) A tattoo before and after 2QS sessions (clinical and dermoscopic picture before any treatment on the left, and after 2 months on the right). (**c**) The software's pigmentary filter highlights the restitution ad integrum in the treated area. (**d**) The software's vascular filter highlights a reduction of the inflammatory response. (Courtesy of Dr. Domenico Piccolo, Skin Center Avezzano, Italy)

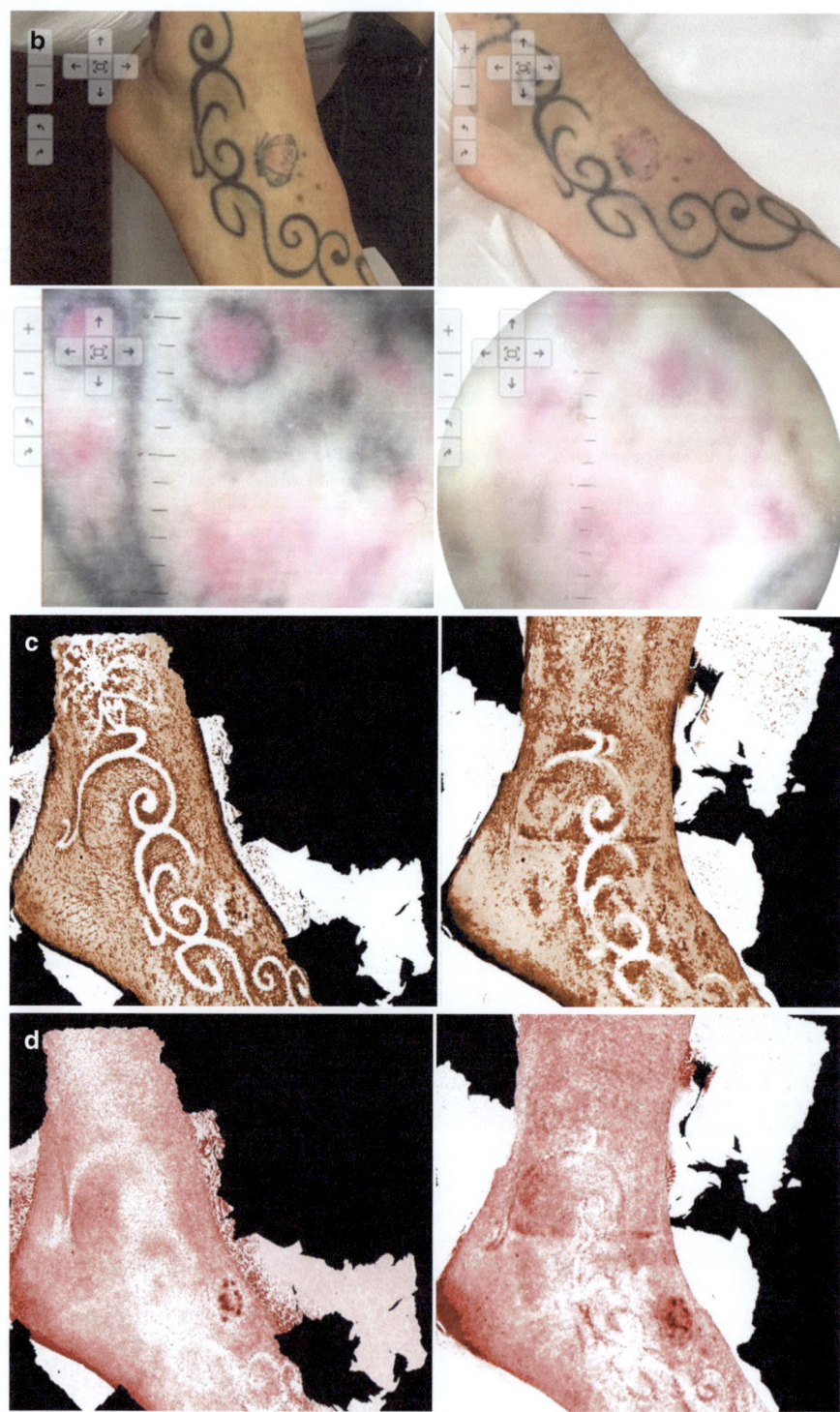

Fig. 12.6 (continued)

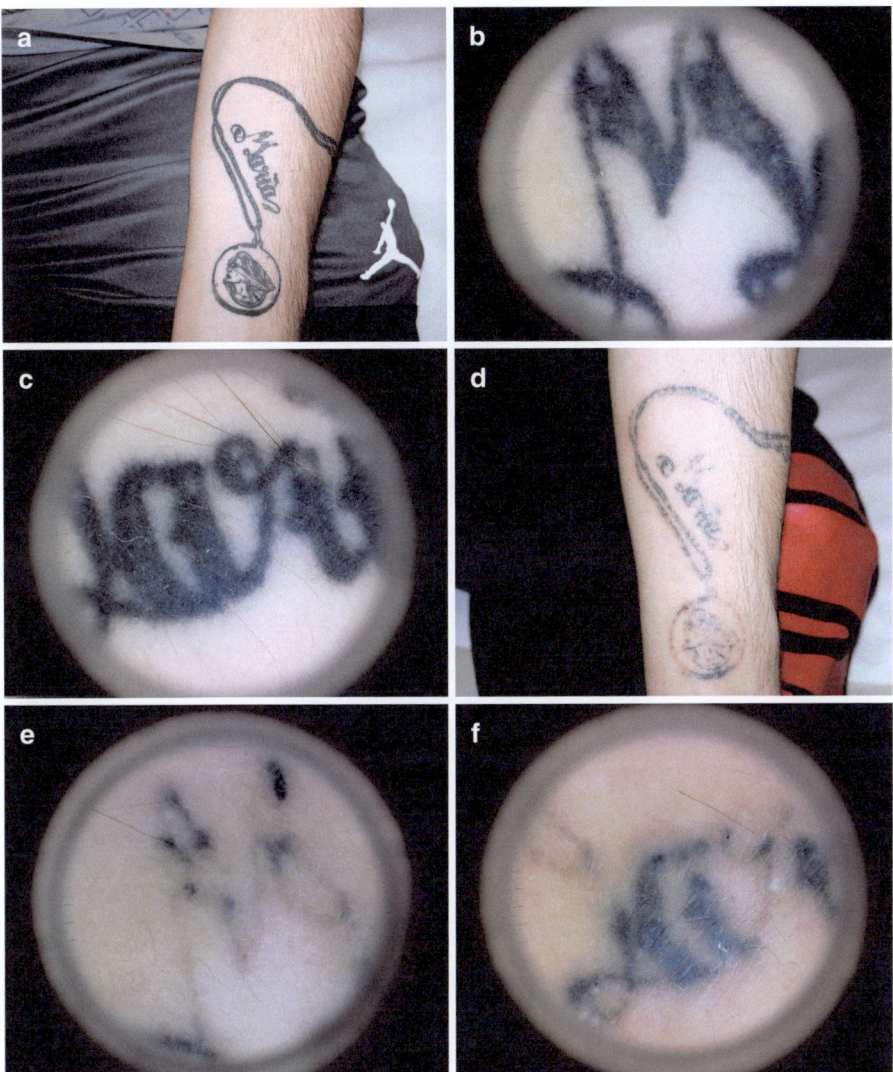

Fig. 12.7 (**a**) Clinical image of a tattoo before any treatment. (**b, c**) Dermoscopic images of the tattoo highlighting the pigment distribution before any treatment. (**d**) Clinical picture of the tattoo after 2QS sessions. (**e, f**) Dermoscopic images of the tattoo highlighting the initial partial destruction of the black pigment after 2QS sessions (courtesy of Dr. Domenico Piccolo, Skin Center Avezzano, Italy). (**g**) Clinical picture of the tattoo after 4QS sessions. (**h, i**) Dermoscopic images of the tattoo highlighting the consistent destruction of the black pigment after 4QS sessions. (**j**) Clinical picture of the tattoo before any treatment on the left and after 7QS sessions on the right. (**k**) Dermoscopic image of the tattoo highlighting the minimal residual of the black pigment after 7QS sessions. (**l**) The software's pigmentary filter highlights the restitution ad integrum in the treated area. (**m**) The software's vascular filter highlights a consistent reduction of the inflammatory response. (Courtesy of Dr. Domenico Piccolo, Skin Center Avezzano, Italy)

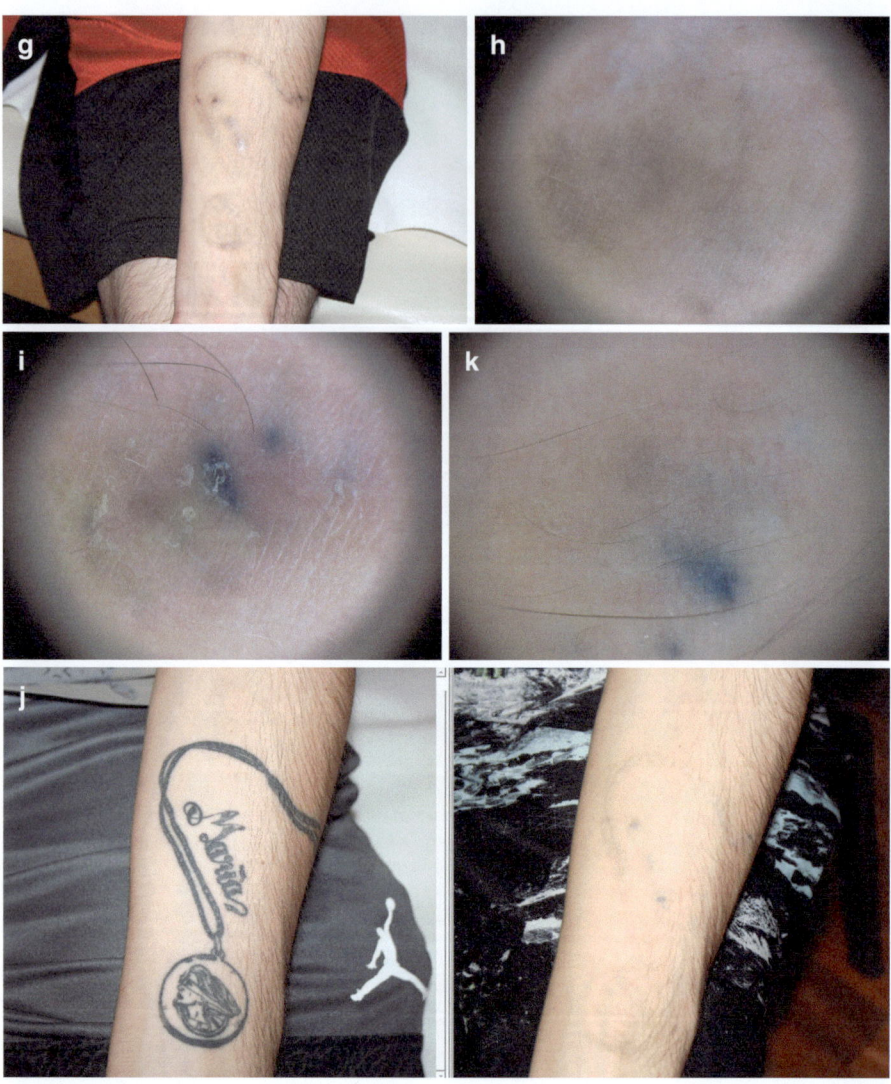

Fig. 12.7 (continued)

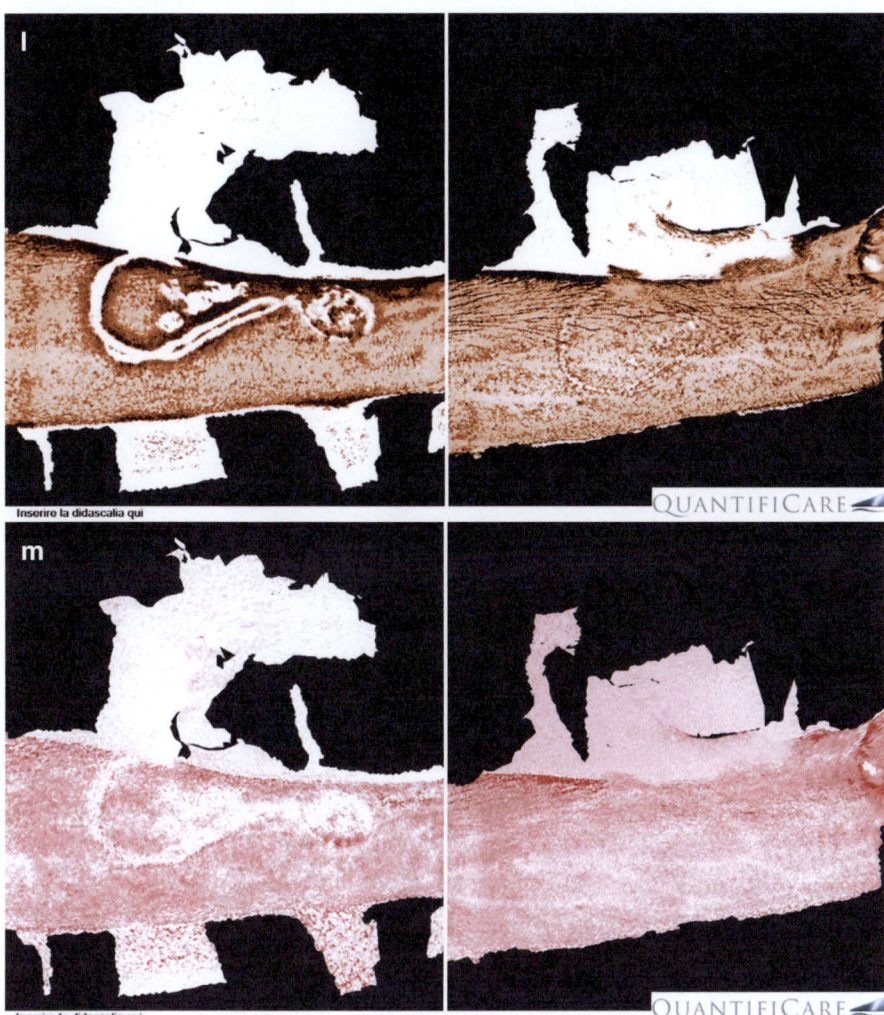

Fig. 12.7   (continued)

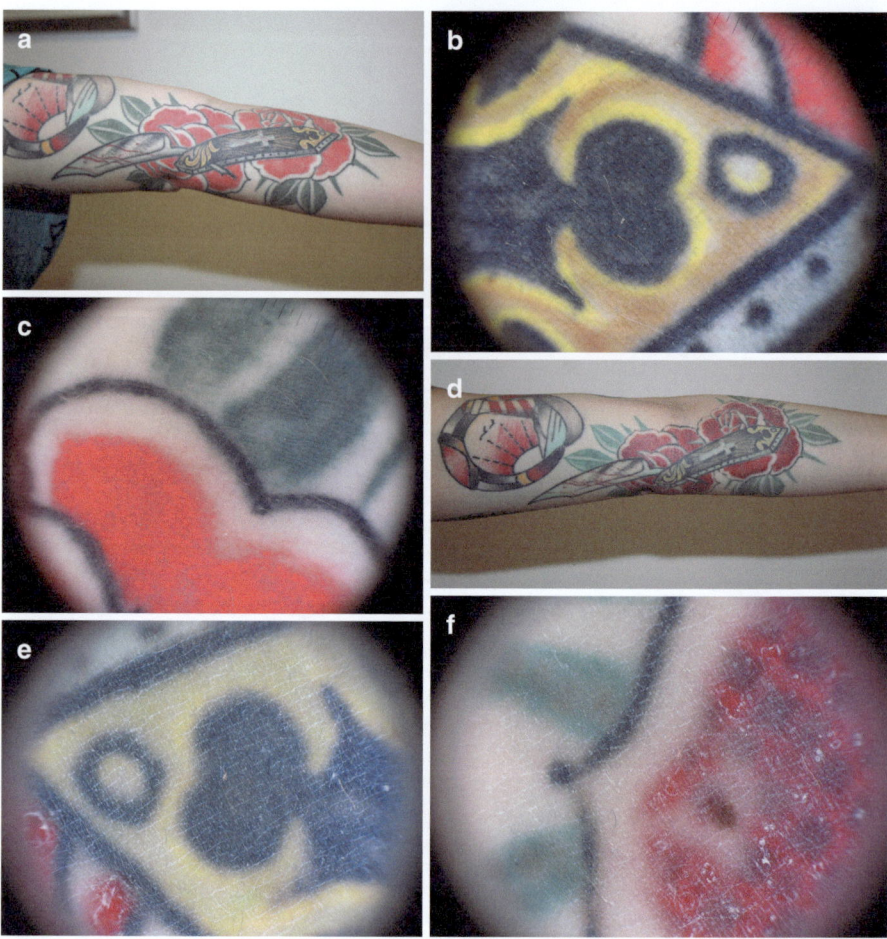

Fig. 12.8 (**a**) Clinical image of a colored tattoo before any treatment. (**b**) Dermoscopic exam of the tattoo highlighting the yellow pigment distribution. (**c**) Dermoscopic exam of the tattoo highlighting the red pigment distribution. (**d**) Clinical picture of the tattoo after 2QS sessions. (**e**) Dermoscopic exam of the tattoo highlighting the initial partial destruction of the yellow pigment after 2QS sessions. (**f**) Dermoscopic exam of the tattoo highlighting the initial partial destruction of the red pigment after 2QS sessions. (**g**) Clinical picture of the tattoo after 4QS sessions. (**h**) Dermoscopic exam of the tattoo highlighting the consistent destruction of the yellow pigment after 4QS sessions. (**i**) Dermoscopic exam of the tattoo highlighting the consistent destruction of the red pigment after 4QS sessions. (Courtesy of Dr. Domenico Piccolo, Skin Center Avezzano, Italy)

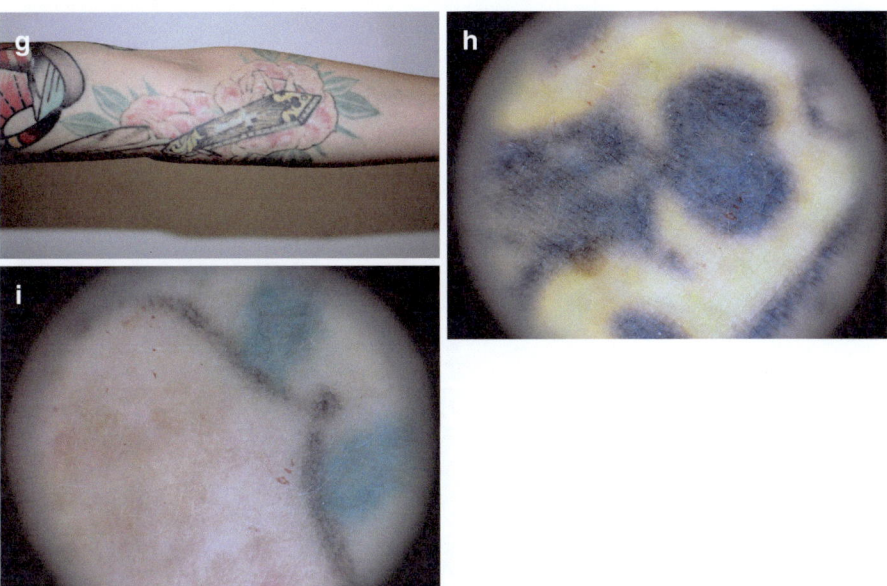

Fig. 12.8 (continued)

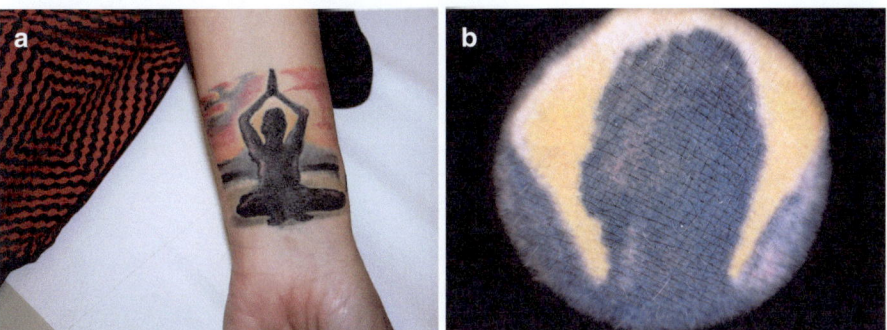

Fig. 12.9 (**a**) Clinical image of a tattoo before any treatment. (**b–d**) Dermoscopic images of the tattoo highlighting the different colored pigments distribution before any treatment. (**e**) Clinical picture of the tattoo before and immediately after 1QS session. (**f**) The software's vascular filter highlights a consistent reduction of the inflammatory response in the treated areas immediately after 1QS session. (**g**) The software's pigmentary filter highlights a consistent reduction of the pigment immediately after 1QS session. (**h**) Clinical picture of the tattoo after 2QS sessions. (**i–k**) Dermoscopic images of the tattoo highlighting the initial partial destruction of the black, yellow, and red pigments at the follow-up visit after 1QS session. (**l**) Clinical picture of the tattoo after 2QS sessions. (**m, n**) Dermoscopic images of the tattoo highlighting the consistent destruction of the black, yellow, and red pigments after 2QS sessions. (**o**) Clinical picture of the tattoo before any treatment on the left and after 2QS sessions on the right. (**p**) The software's vascular filter highlights a consistent reduction of the inflammatory response. (**q**) The software's pigmentary filter highlights a consistent reduction of the pigment in the treated areas. (Courtesy of Dr. Domenico Piccolo, Skin Center Avezzano, Italy)

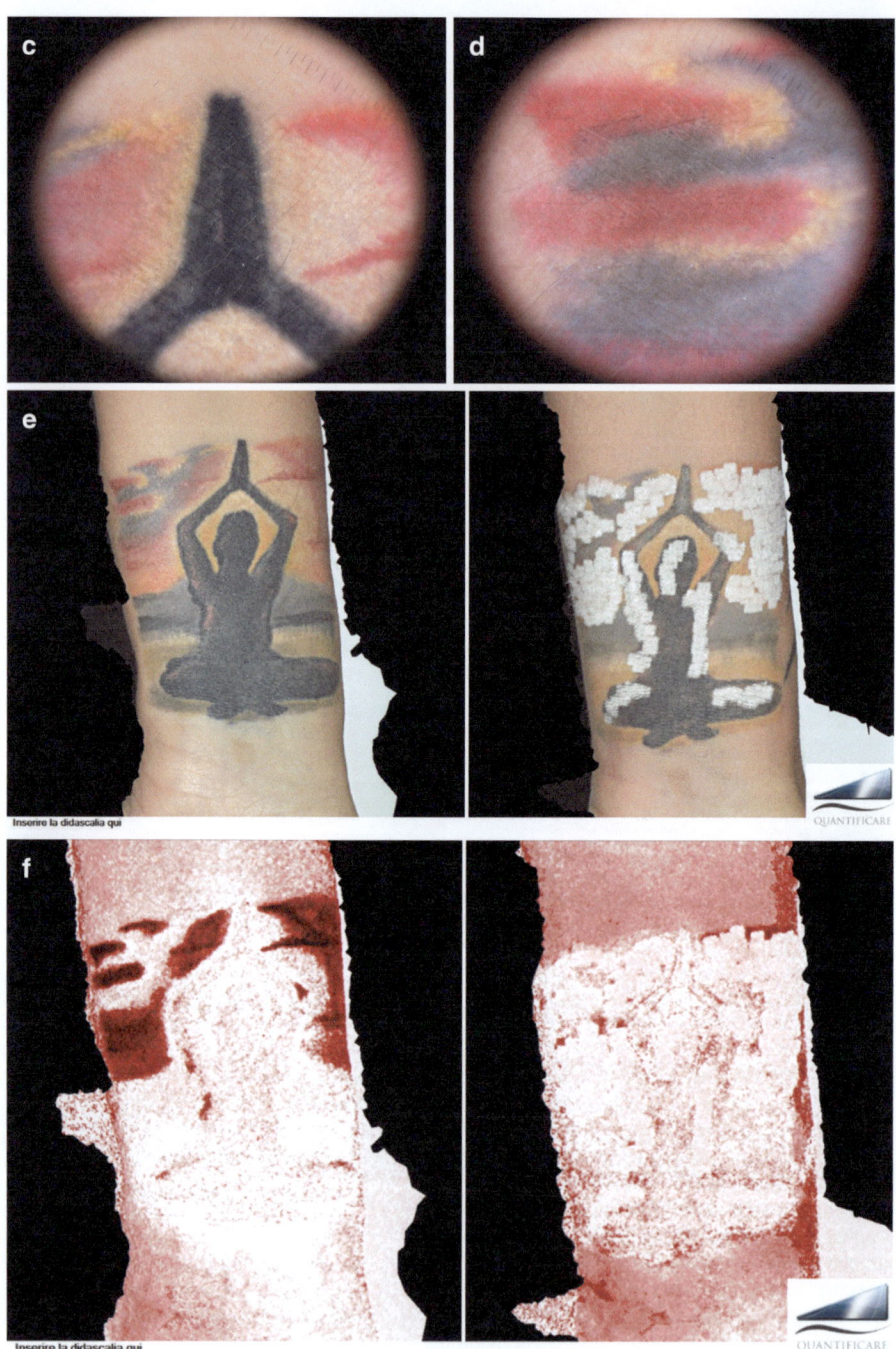

Inserire la didascalia qui

Inserire la didascalia qui

Fig. 12.9 (continued)

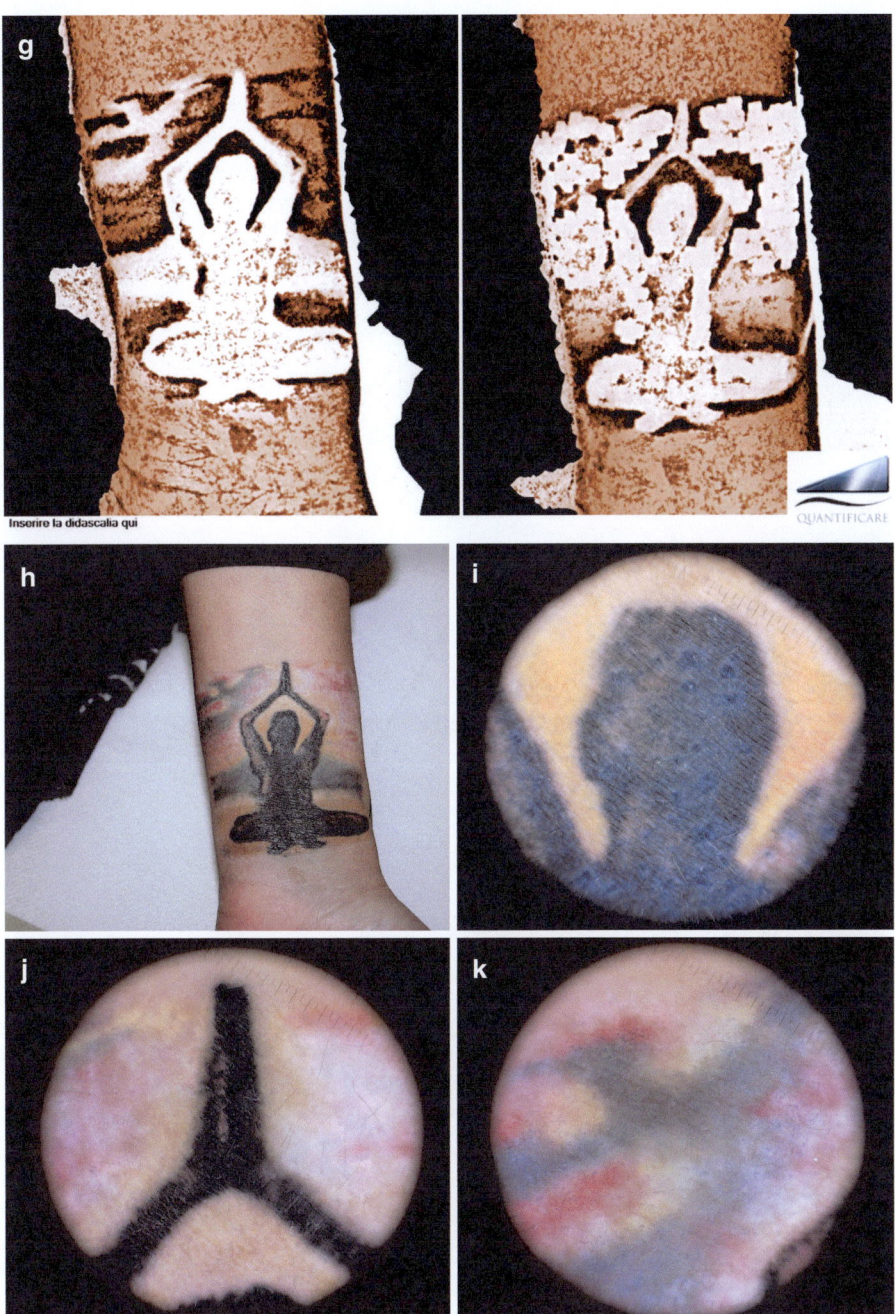

Inserire la didascalia qui

Fig. 12.9 (continued)

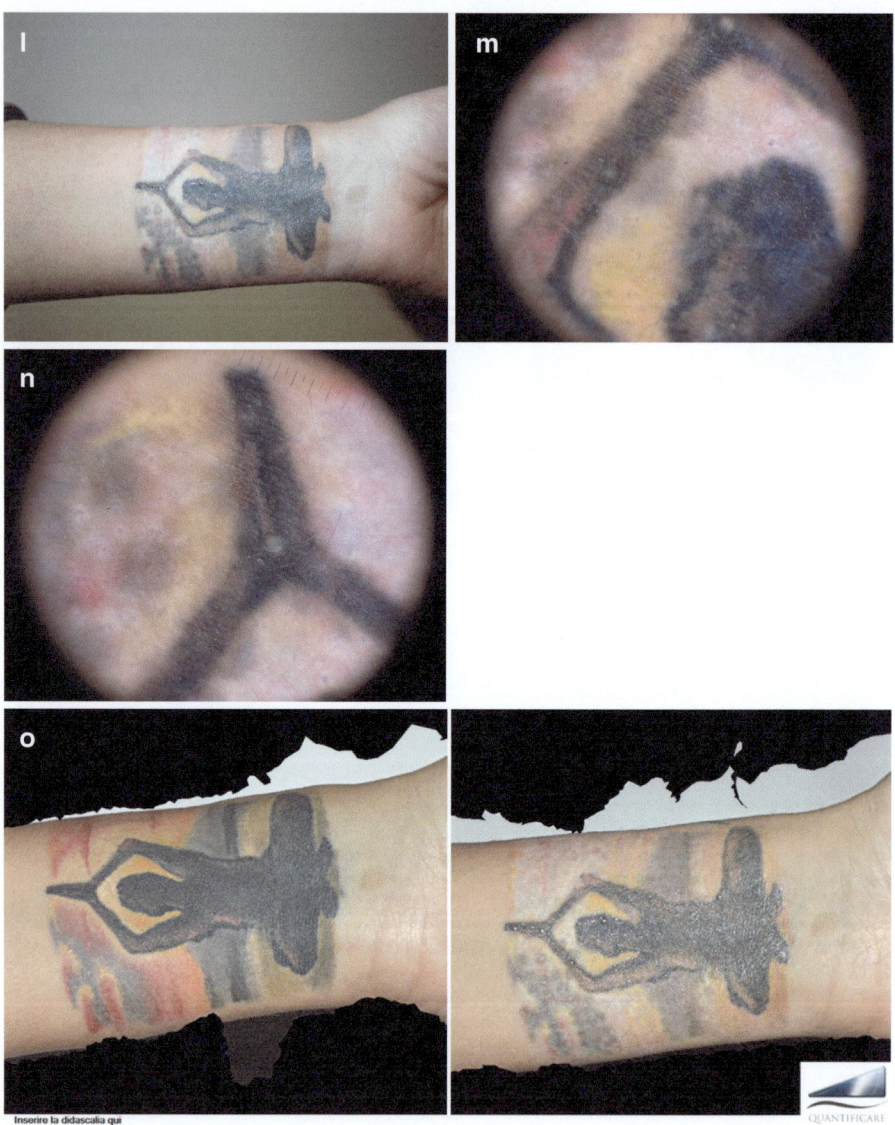

Fig. 12.9 (continued)

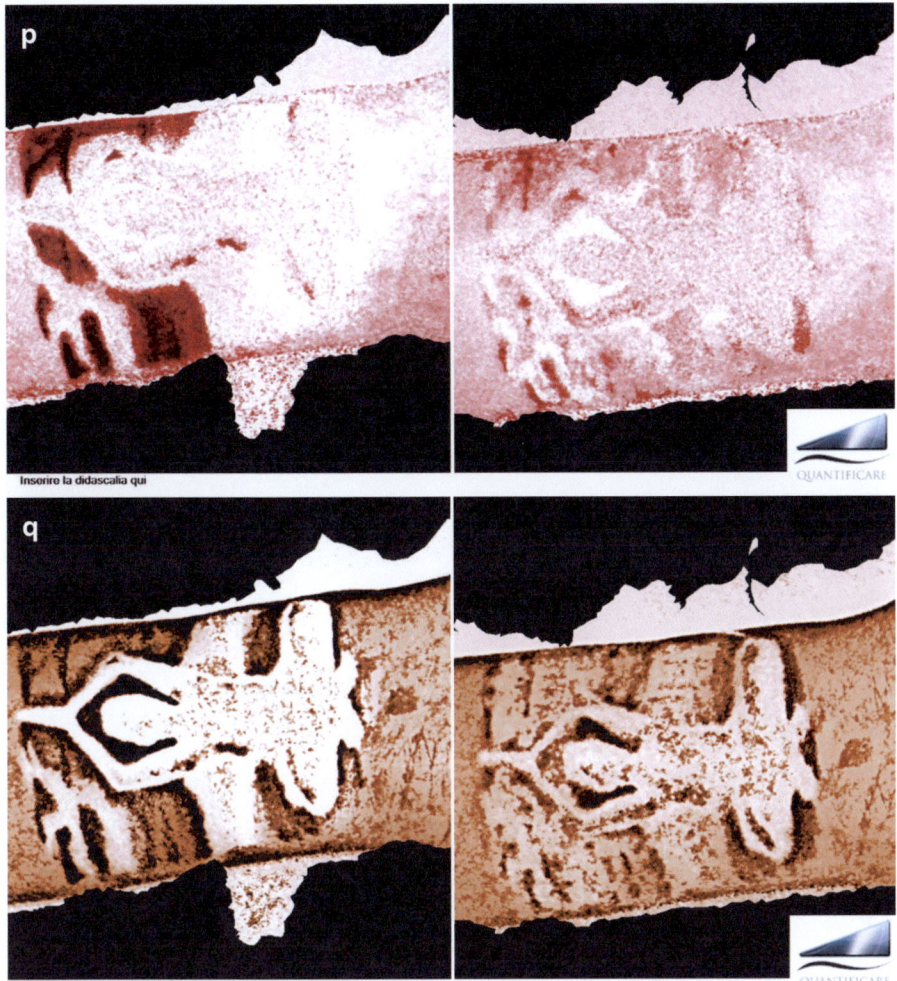

Inserire la didascalia qui

Inserire la didascalia qui

Fig. 12.9 (continued)

References

Antoszewski B, Sitek A, Fijałkowska M, et al. Tattooing and body piercing--what motivates you to do it? Int J Soc Psychiatry. 2010;56:471–9.

Arbache S, Roth D, Arbache ST, et al. Original method to repigment achromic laser tattoo removal scars. Case Rep Dermatol. 2019;11(2):140–4.

Bassi A, Campolmi P, Cannarozzo G, et al. Tattoo-associated skin reaction: the importance of an early diagnosis and proper treatment. Biomed Res Int. 2014;2014:354608.

Carmen R, Guitar A, Dillon H. Ultimate answers to proximate questions: the evolutionary motivations behind tattoos and body piercings in popular culture. Rev Gen Psychol. 2012;16:134–43.

Dickson L, Dukes R, Smith H, et al. To ink or not to ink: the meaning of tattoos among college students. Coll Stud J. 2015;49:106–20.

Fulton JE Jr, Rahimi AD, Mansoor S, et al. The treatment of hypopigmentation after skin resurfacing. Dermatol Surg. 2004;30(1):95–101.

Glassy C, Glassy M, Aldasoiuqi A. Tattooing: medical uses and problems. Cleve Clin J Med. 2012;79:761–70.

Grimm S, Cronin A. Health risks associated with tattoos and body piercing. J Clin Outcomes Manag. 2014;21:315–6.

Kaur RR, Kirby W, Mailbach H. Cutaneous allergic reactions to tattoo ink. J Cosmet Dermatol. 2009;8:295–300.

Kierstein L, Kjelskau KC. Tattoo as art, the drivers behind the fascination and the decision to become tattooed. Curr Probl Dermatol. 2015;48:37–40.

Kirby W, Desai A, Desai T, et al. The Kirby-Desai scale: a proposed scale to assess tattoo-removal treatments. J Clin Aesthet Dermatol. 2009;2(3):32–7.

Rahimi IA, Eberhard I, Kasten E. TATTOOS: what do people really know about the medical risks of body ink? J Clin Aesthet Dermatol. 2018;11:30–5.

Dermoscopy Applied to PDT with IPL Treatments: Nonmelanoma Skin Cancers

13

13.1 Nonmelanoma Skin Cancers (NMSCs)

Nonmelanoma skin cancers (NMSCs), namely actinic keratosis, basal cell carcinoma, Bowen's disease, and squamous cell carcinoma, are slow-growing skin tumors that are characterized by low risk of metastatic potential and favorable prognosis and represent the most common malignancy among the Caucasian population (Babilas et al. 2007). Over the last decades, the worldwide incidence is estimated to rise by 3–10% (Palm and Goldman 2011), presenting an increasing demand on healthcare resources.

13.2 Treatment Options (Courtesy of Dr. Domenico Piccolo— Skin Center Avezzano, Italy)

Surgery has been the "gold standard" treatment for years. Thanks to a precise identification of the tumor margins, it provides high rates of disease control, even though conservative therapies should be considered, based on lesion characteristics (location and size, particularly for AK, sBCC, and BD) as well as patient-specific factors (age, comorbidity, medications, immunosuppression) (Wan and Lin 2014).

The surgical technique of Mohs (also called chemosurgery or microscopically controlled surgery) was introduced in 1938 by Frederic E. Mohs for the microscopic treatment of common types of skin cancer. It consists of the intraoperative microscopic examination by the surgeon of each portion of tissue removed during surgery; this allows the identification of the neoplasm and the margins of excision. The second information suggests to the surgeon which and how much tissue to remove later. It is one of the methods used to obtain complete control of the margins during skin cancer removal procedures using physical (cold) or chemical histological techniques (through the use of fixatives and dyes).

The contents of this book are partially based on the Italian language edition: *"The Usefulness of Dermoscopy in Laser and IPL Treatments"*, Domenico Piccolo, © DEKA M.E.L.A Srl 2012.

© Springer Nature Switzerland AG 2020

D. Piccolo et al., *Quick Guide to Dermoscopy in Laser and IPL Treatments*, https://doi.org/10.1007/978-3-319-41633-5_13

Success rates with Mohs surgery take on different percentages based on the skin lesion involved: from 99.8% of success rate in the treatment of basal cell carcinoma and 94% of success rate in the treatment of squamous cell carcinoma, to 77–98% of success rate in the treatment of melanoma in situ (depending on surgeons' ability) and 52% of success rate in the treatment of other types of malignant melanoma.

Photodynamic therapy (PDT) with topical 5-aminolevulinic acid (ALA) or methyl aminolevulinate (MAL) has proven to be a highly effective conservative method for the treatment of AK, sBCC, and BD, with the benefit of excellent cosmetic results and the potential for field treatment (Ruiz-Rodriguez et al. 2002).

The rationale for using the IPL as a light source for PDT is based on the absorption spectrum of the photosensitizer and IPL's features. Protoporphyrin IX (PpIX) has absorption peaks at 505, 540, 580, and 630 nm. IPL is a source of incoherent light with emission spectrum ranging from 500 to 1200 nm. By using different cut-off filters in the handpiece, the delivered wavelengths can be varied, underlying IPL's versatility. Thus, the adaptation to the absorption spectrum of PpIX allows for the use of IPL for PDT (Palm and Goldman 2011).

In 2008, in a controlled prospective study by Tadiparthi et al. (2008), MAL-IPL has also been found to be more effective in treating large areas of AK than IPL alone; however, the AK clearance rate after MAL-IPL was slightly higher than the AK clearance rate after IPL alone (60% versus 55%).

In 2009, Downs et al. (2009) evaluated the efficacy of MAL-PDT using an IPL in 40 patients with mixed diagnoses, including AK (11 lesions of the scalp and ten in different sites), BD (9), and sBCC (10). In terms of BD and sBCC outcomes, a 100% clearance rate was reached at 4 months after treatment. The complete clearance rate for scalp and various AKs was 91% and 100%, respectively. Only a partial recurrence was observed in an immunocompromised patient. All patients experienced heat and mild to moderate pain that lasted for less than a second.

According to the literature, the efficacy of IPL-PDT in BD and sBCC is based only on small series of cases. Hasegawa et al. (2010) treated three patients who were clinically and histopathologically diagnosed with BD. All patients were treated with ALA-PDT by IPL. Five sessions were performed with 2-week intervals. After treatment, all patients experienced mild transient edema, erythema, scaling, and healing crusts within 10 days. No clinical signs of relapse were observed at 1-year follow-up.

So far there are no treatment parameters defined for the use of IPL in PDT. Haddad et al. (2011) compared several doses of IPL light for ALA-PDT of AK and photodamaged skin and showed that a greater fluidity of IPL leads to a better AK result, but not an increase in photodamage improvement.

A recent prospective randomized, placebo-controlled study by Kohl et al. (Kohl 2017) evaluated the efficacy of MAL-PDT with IPL compared to placebo-IPL for the treatment of dorsal AK. At the 10-week follow-up, complete AK clearance rates per hand were 54.5% after MAL-IPL and 3.0% after placebo-IPL ($p < 0.0001$) while complete AK clearance rates for lesions were respectively 69% and 15% ($p < 0.001$). Both treatment modalities significantly improved the photodamaged skin of the dorsal hands and induced neocollagenesis.

Piccolo D. and Kostaki D. published in 2018 their results with a PDT-IPL therapy in a group of 25 patients, with a total of 29 lesions, including AK (20), sBCC

(5), and BD (4). All patients had large, multiple lesions in aesthetically sensitive areas and therefore did not represent ideal candidates for surgical therapy. Dermoscopy proved to be fundamental for the diagnosis of most lesions, while in doubtful cases biopsy was used to rule out the correct diagnosis with the histological examination.

All hyperkeratotic lesions were first treated with CO_2 laser to increase the penetration of cream and light. MAL (Metvix®, Galderma Italia S.p.A, Agrate Brianza, Italy) was applied to the lesion as a 1 mm thick layer, including 5 mm of surrounding normal tissue, while if multiple lesions occurred it was applied over the entire anatomical area. A nonabsorbent occlusive shell was placed over the MAL to increase its penetration, and an aluminum sheet was positioned above to eliminate exposure to light. After 3 h occlusion, MAL was removed, a thin layer of chilled gel was applied, and irradiation was performed.

IPL has been set with the following parameters: cut-off wavelength, 550 nm; fluence, 18 J/cm²; triple pulse mode (first pulse of 3.3 nm, second pulse of 4.6 ms, and the third one of 2.1 ms in duration); interpulse delay, 100 ms with epidermal cooling already provided by the IPL handpiece.

Actinic keratoses (Fig. 13.1a, b) required three passages of irradiation in a single treatment session (Fig. 13.1c, d), while sBCC and BD lesions required four passages of irradiation in two treatment sessions at 2-week intervals. Patients reported only mild pain during irradiation of the lesion and slight heat after treatment for less than 20 s. Transient edema and erythema occurred after each session, followed by crusting with healing within 1 week. Post-treatment care included a topical antibacterial ointment and a sunscreen cream, and patients were strictly advised to avoid sunlight and to use sunscreen for the following 6 weeks. This study of Piccolo D. and Kostaki D. demonstrated a complete clinical and dermoscopic response in 18 of the 20 AKs (90%) (Fig. 13.1e, f), and partial response in the rest (10%), and a complete response in 4/5 sBCC (80%) and in 4/4 BD (100%), while partial response was observed in 1/5 sBCC (20%). In conclusion, they obtained a clinical and dermoscopic resolution in 26 of 29 lesions (89.6%) after one or two IPL-PDT sessions, according to the treatment protocol. At the 5-year follow-up, the cosmetic result was excellent in 29 out of 29 (100%).

13.3   The Validity of Dermoscopy in the Treatment of NMSCs

The validity of dermoscopy in the treatment of nonmelanoma skin cancers with PDT (with or without IPL) is widely demonstrated. In particular, dermoscopy is indispensable to highlight the typical characteristics of basal cell carcinomas such as arborizing vessels, leaf-like areas, gray-blue ovoid nests, gray-blue dots and globules, and spoked-wheels areas (Figs. 13.2a, b, 13.3, and 13.4a, b).

The dermoscopic examination performed a few days after the treatment shows a complete or partial disappearance of the diagnostic patterns (Figs. 13.2c, d, 13.3, and 13.4c, d).

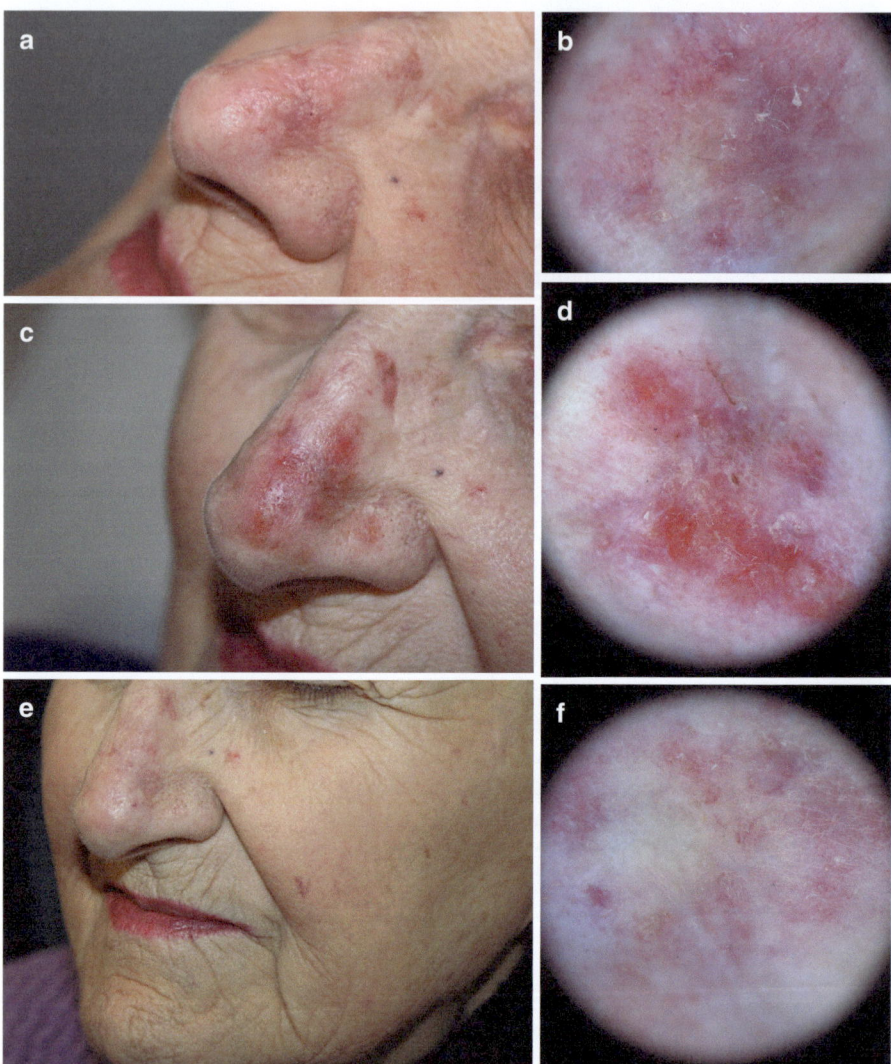

Fig. 13.1 (**a**) Clinical picture of actinic keratosis of the nose in an old woman before any treatment. (**b**) Dermoscopy performed before any treatment is mandatory to rule out the correct diagnosis; an actinic keratosis has been confirmed in this case. (**c**) Clinical image taken immediately after one session of PDT active by IPL. (**d**) The dermoscopic exam performed immediately after treatment reveals the color change from pink to red. (**e**) Clinical image after two PDT sessions activated by IPL. (**f**) The excellent clinical results are confirmed at the dermoscopy with the complete clearance of the lesion. (Courtesy of Dr. Domenico Piccolo, Skin Center Avezzano, Italy)

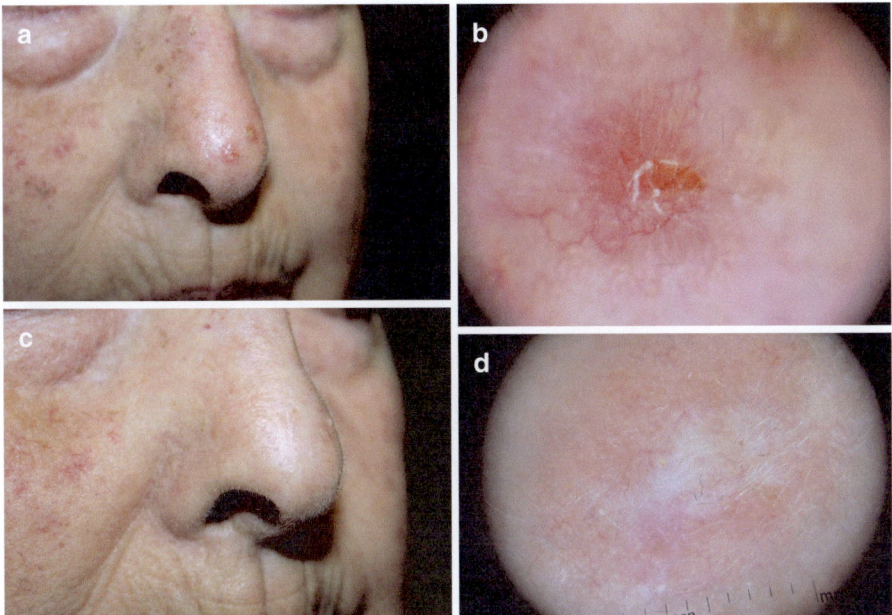

Fig. 13.2 (**a**) Clinical picture of a basal cell carcinoma of the nose in an old woman before any treatment. (**b**) Dermoscopy performed before any treatment demonstrated the presence of arborizing vessels and ulceration. (**c**) Clinical image after two PDT sessions activated by IPL. (**d**) The excellent clinical results are confirmed at the dermoscopy with the complete clearance of the lesion. (Courtesy of Dr. Domenico Piccolo, Skin Center Avezzano, Italy)

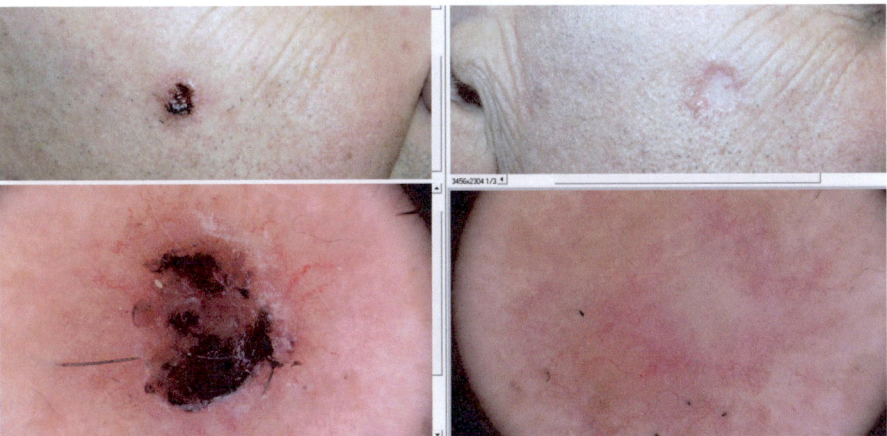

Fig. 13.3 Clinical and dermoscopic images of an ulcerated basal cell carcinoma of the cheek in an old man, successfully treated with PDT with IPL. (Courtesy of Dr. Domenico Piccolo, Skin Center Avezzano, Italy)

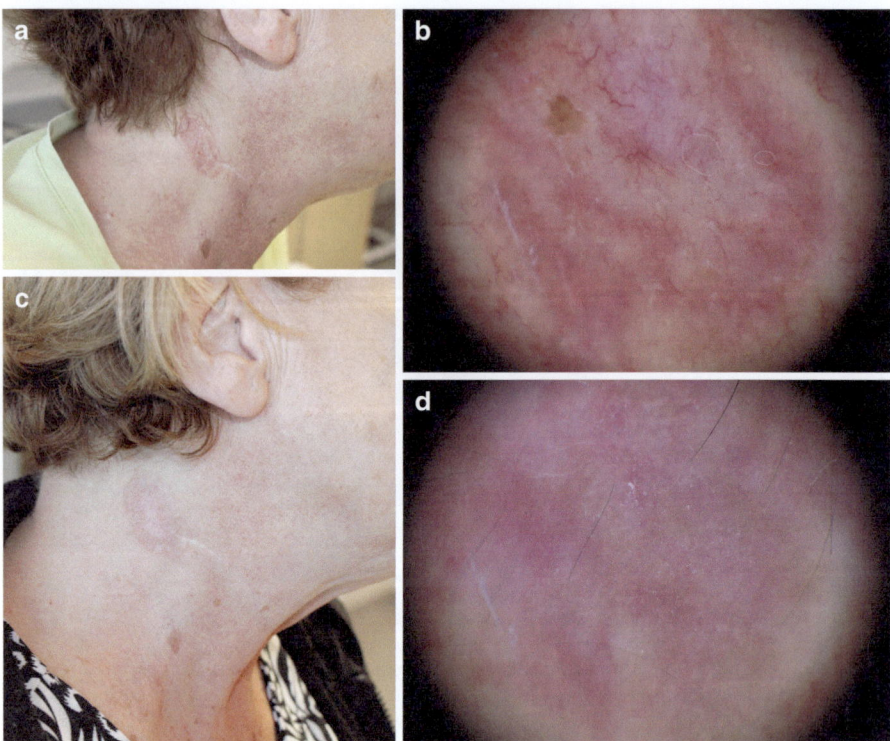

Fig. 13.4 (**a**) Clinical picture of a basal cell carcinoma on the neck in an old woman before any treatment. (**b**) Dermoscopy performed before any treatment demonstrated the presence of arborizing vessels and ulceration. (**c**) Clinical image after two CO_2 laser and one PDT session activated by IPL. (**d**) The excellent clinical results are confirmed at the dermoscopy with the complete clearance of the lesion. (Courtesy of Dr. Domenico Piccolo, Skin Center Avezzano, Italy)

References

Babilas P, Knobler R, Hummel S, et al. Variable pulsed light is less painful than light- emitting diodes for topical photodynamic therapy of actinic keratosis: a prospective randomized controlled trial. Br J Dermatol. 2007;157:111–7.

Downs AM, Bower CB, Oliver DA, et al. Methyl aminolaevulinate-photodynamic therapy for actinic keratoses, squamous cell carcinoma in situ and superficial basal cell carcinoma employing a square wave intense pulsed light device for photoactivation. Br J Dermatol. 2009;161:189–90.

Haddad A, Santos ID, Gragnani A, et al. The effect of increasing fluence on the treatment of actinic keratosis and photodamage by photodynamic therapy with 5-aminolevulinic acid and intense pulsed light. Photomed Laser Surg. 2011;29:427–32.

Hasegawa T, Suga Y, Mizuno Y, et al. Efficacy of photodynamic therapy with topical 5-aminolevulinic acid using intense pulsed light for Bowen's disease. J Dermatol. 2010;37:623–8.

Kohl E, Popp C, Zeman F, et al. Photodynamic therapy using intense pulsed light for treating actinic keratoses and photoaged skin of the dorsal hands: a randomized placebo-controlled study. Br J Dermatol. 2017;176(2):352–62.

Palm M, Goldman PM. Aminolevulinic acid: actinic keratosis and photorejuvenation. In: Gold MH, editor. Photodynamic therapy in dermatology. New York, NY: Springer Science and Business Media, LLC; 2011. p. 5–30. ISBN 978-1-4419-1297-8.

Piccolo D, Kostaki D. Photodynamic therapy activated by intense pulsed light in the treatment of nonmelanoma skin cancer. Biomedicine. 2018;6(1):E18.

Ruiz-Rodriguez R, Sanz-Sánchez T, Córdoba S. Photodynamic Photorejuvenation. Dermatol Surg. 2002;28(8):742–44.

Tadiparthi S, Falder S, Saour S, et al. Intense pulsed light with methyl-aminolevulinic acid for the treatment of actinic keratoses. Plast Reconstr Surg. 2008;121:351e–2e.

Wan MT, Lin JT. Current evidence and applications of photodynamic therapy in dermatology. Clin Cosmet Investig Dermatol. 2014;21:145–63.

The Validity of Dermoscopy in Determining Any Adverse Effects

Adverse effects may occur after any treatment with laser or IPL and may depend on patient's overreaction or on the incorrect choice of the used devices or on an inappropriate parameters' setting selected by the clinician.

Recently, Jalian et al. (2013) reported the most common causes of legal action related to various cutaneous laser surgeries from 1985 to 2012. It was found that the first cause is related to thermal burns, while "scarring" (which included hypertrophic scars and keloids) comprised nearly 39% of injuries sustained secondary to laser treatments from various devices. As a matter of fact, side effects can occur.

As reported recently by Thaysen-Petersen et al. (2017), IPL induced a wide range of skin reactions, including erythema (87% of the 16 enrolled subjects), purpura (27%), blisters (20%), edema (13%), crusting (13%), hyperpigmentation (60%), and hypopigmentation (20%). They reported that skin pigmentation (the darker the skin the higher risk of adverse effects) and increasing IPL fluence represent the major determinants for IPL-induced side effects.

Lasers adverse effects encountered:

- Dyspigmentation (hypopigmentation, which may resolve spontaneously with repigmentation after a few months; hyperpigmentation, which can subsequently be treated with IPL) (Figs. 14.1 and 14.2)
- Aberrant cicatricial reactions, even reported as rare events (Kluger et al. 2009; Goldstein 1979) such as hypertrophic or keloids following inappropriate laser treatment (CO_2 laser) or appropriate laser treatment (QS) but with an individual aberrant response (Fig. 14.3a, b)
- Blistering
- Crusting

The contents of this book are partially based on the Italian language edition: "*The Usefulness of Dermoscopy in Laser and IPL Treatments*", Domenico Piccolo, © DEKA M.E.L.A Srl 2012.

© Springer Nature Switzerland AG 2020
D. Piccolo et al., *Quick Guide to Dermoscopy in Laser and IPL Treatments*, https://doi.org/10.1007/978-3-319-41633-5_14

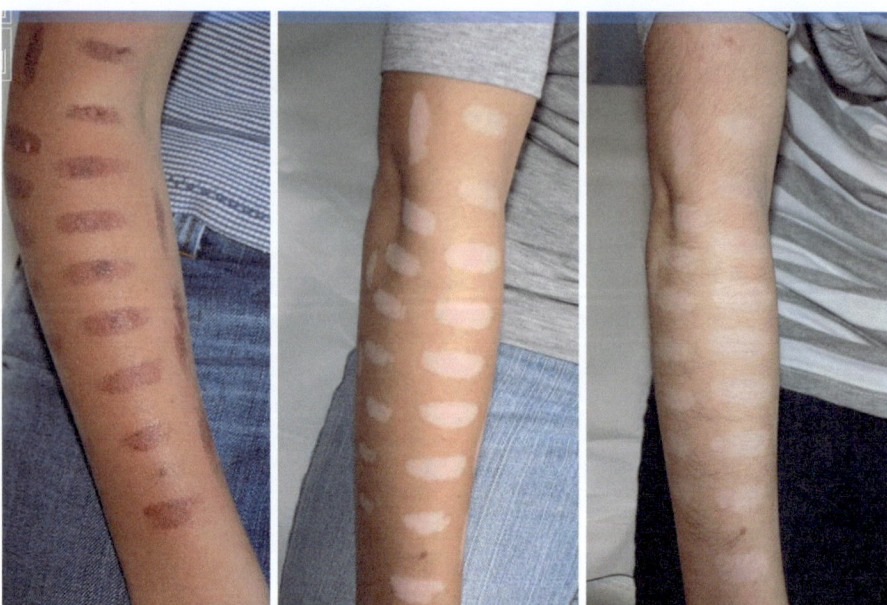

Fig. 14.1 Hyperpigmentation and hypopigmentation after an IPL session for hair removal. (Courtesy of Dr. Domenico Piccolo, Skin Center Avezzano, Italy)

Fig. 14.2 Hyperpigmentation after a Nd:YAG session for hair removal. (Courtesy of Dr. Domenico Piccolo, Skin Center Avezzano, Italy)

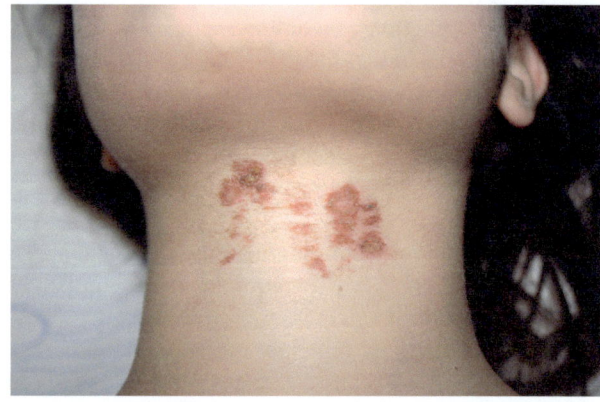

In our experience, dermoscopy has proven to be an extraordinary tool to determine any adverse effects immediately after a laser or IPL treatment. This allows the doctor to provide adequate therapy in advance and to inform the patient about any side effects.

As previously reported in this text, the change in color from brown to gray can be considered a prodromic sign of therapeutic success in treating benign pigmented lesions. On the other side, the change in shape with the removal of the pigment can be clearly detected with dermoscopy and represents an indication of immediate damage to the skin.

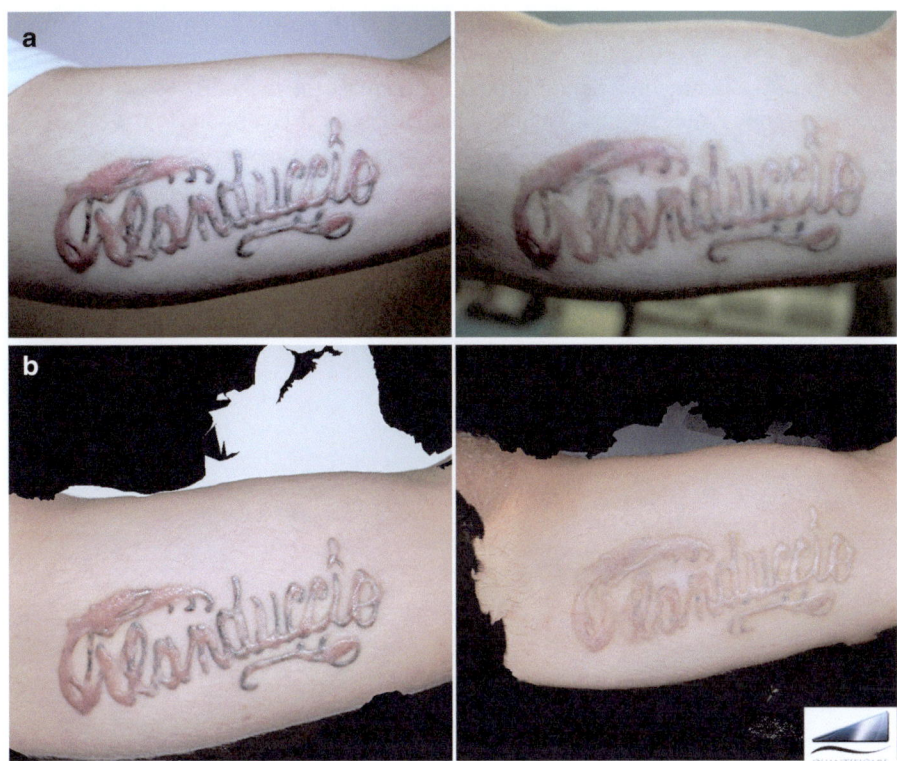

Inserire la didascalia qui

Fig. 14.3 (**a**) Keloid after a QS laser session for tattoo removal. The laser was appropriate for the intent, but the individual response was aberrant. (**b**) Clinical improvement after two sessions with dye laser and then QS again. (Courtesy of Dr. Domenico Piccolo, Skin Center Avezzano, Italy)

One month after the treatment, this damage usually generates complete destruction of the pigmentation, resulting in the disappearance of the treated lesion, but with the subsequent appearance of a hypopigmented and erythematous area, composed of the presence of a fine telangiectasias at the dermoscopic exam.

A few months later, a complete repigmentation of the treated area has been documented.

Dermoscopy is also useful to determine the adverse effect resulting from other events, and it is fundamental to select the appropriate corrective treatment.

We report on the case of a young woman (Fitzpatrick III) presented with post-inflammatory hyperpigmentation occurred after a wax and a subsequent aesthetic lamp (Fig. 14.4a). We tested IPL on a little hyperpigmented area in order to verify the good response to the treatment (Fig. 14.4b). The dermoscopic examination that was performed before treatment in order to confirm the hyperpigmenation, and after the IPL treatment thus confirming a clearance of the hyperpigmentation (Fig. 14.4c, d) and highlightening an excellent clinical outcome (Fig. 14.4e).

In another case, a young woman presented with post-inflammatory hyperpigmentation after waxing the eyebrows and subsequent tattooing (Fig. 14.5a). Dermoscopy examination demonstrated an increase in melanin (Fig. 14.5b). An excellent clinical outcome has been reached after one IPL session (Fig. 14.5c, d).

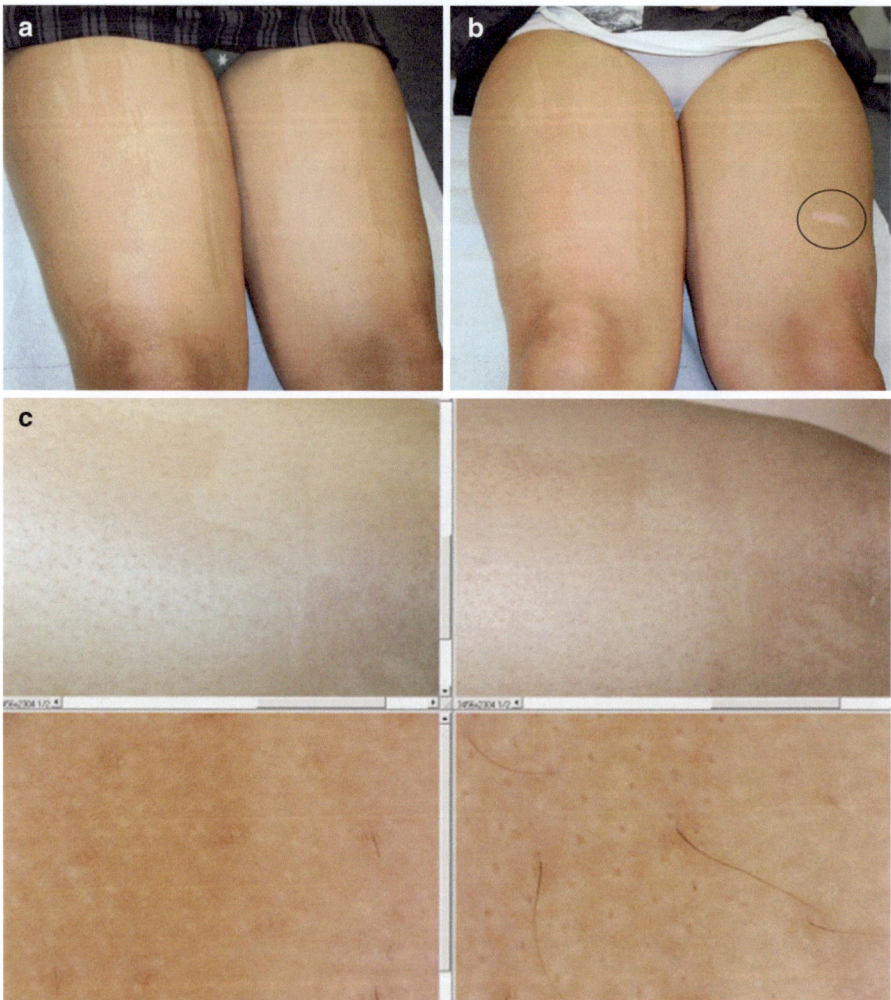

Fig. 14.4 (**a**) Post-inflammatory hyperpigmentation occurred in a Fitzpatrick III young girl after waxing and an aesthetic lamp. (**b**) IPL test on the hyperpigmented area in order to verify the good response to the treatment. (**c**) Before and after an IPL treatment with dermoscopic exam, which confirmed a clearance of the hyperpigmentation. (**d**) Before and after an IPL treatment with dermoscopic exam, which confirmed a clearance of the hyperpigmentation. (**e**) Clinical image of the excellent clinical outcome. (Courtesy of Dr. Domenico Piccolo, Skin Center Avezzano, Italy)

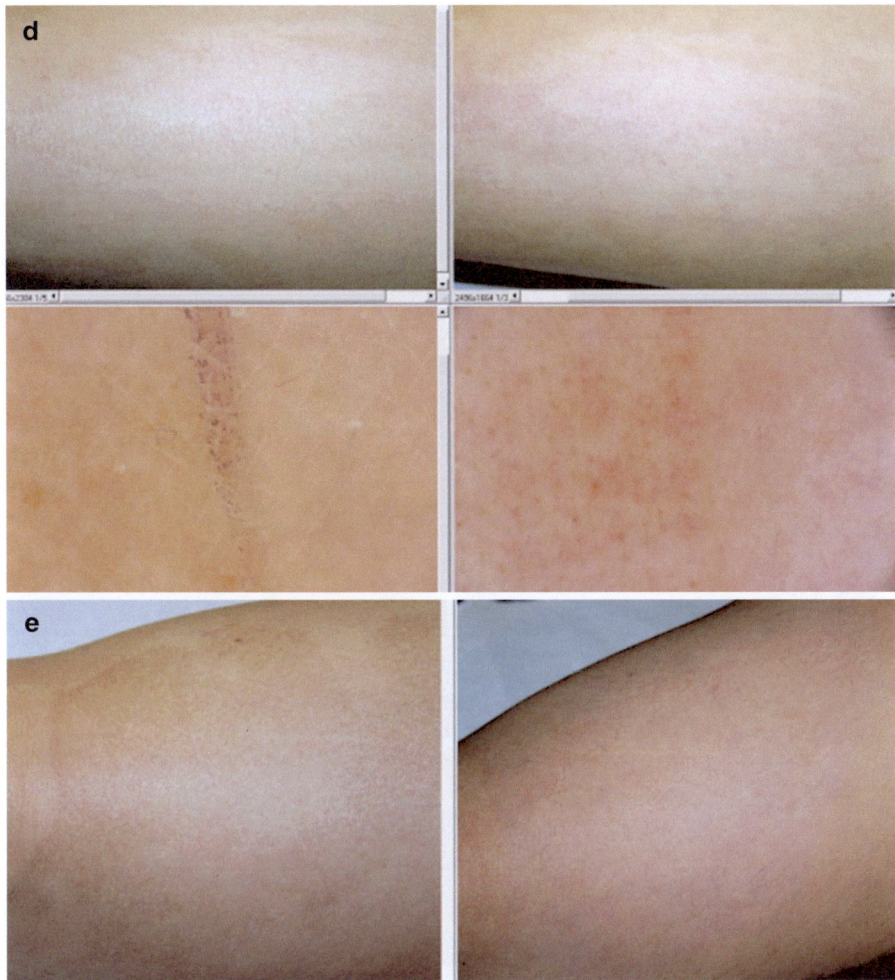

Fig. 14.4 (continued)

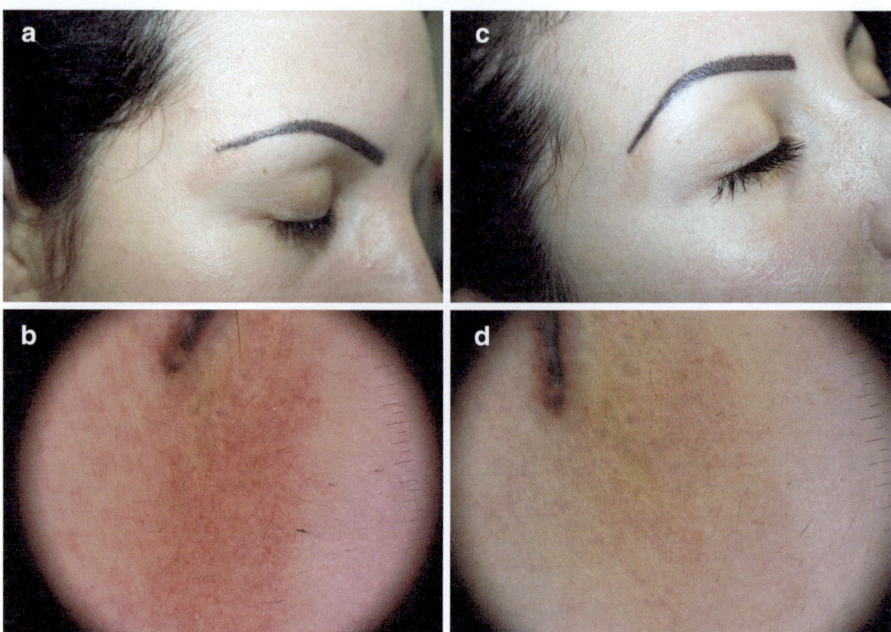

Fig. 14.5 (**a**) Post-inflammatory hyperpigmentation of the eyebrows in a young girl after waxing and subsequent tattooing. (**b**) Dermoscopy exam demonstrated an increase in melanin. (**c**) An excellent clinical outcome has been reached after one IPL session. (**d**) Dermoscopic exam confirming the clearance of the hyperpigmentation. (Courtesy of Dr. Domenico Piccolo, Skin Center Avezzano, Italy)

References

Goldstein N IV. Complications from tattoos. J Dermatol Surg Oncol. 1979;5:869–78.

Jalian HR, Jalian CA, Avram MM. Common causes of injury and legal action in laser surgery. JAMA Dermatol. 2013;149(2):188–93.

Kluger N, Hakimi S, Del Giudice P. Keloid occurring in a tattoo after laser hair removal. Acta Derm Venereol. 2009;89(3):334–5.

Thaysen-Petersen D, Erlendsson AM, Nash JF, et al. Side effects from intense pulsed light: importance of skin pigmentation, fluence level and ultraviolet radiation-a randomized controlled trial. Lasers Surg Med. 2017;49(1):88–96.

Conclusions

15

In our over 20-year clinical experience, dermoscopy represents a useful, effective, and easy-to-use tool for diagnostic and follow-up activities.

With the advent of new laser and pulsed light methodologies in the treatment of the most common dermatological diseases, not only a tool was needed that would allow to formulate the correct diagnostic hypothesis, fundamental for the choice of the therapeutic protocol to be implemented, but also an instrument that was able to objectively evaluate the starting state and the result obtained for each treatment. Until then, this role was entrusted to simple "before and after treatment" clinical photographs, which, however, had the limitation of highlighting only great results, without being able to appreciate the minimum, sometimes microscopic changes between one treatment session and another.

In our clinical practice, we have decided to test dermoscopy as a diagnostic and follow-up tool for all our patients and we have established a strict protocol in order to scientifically validate this method.

As mentioned before, dermoscopic digital images of all patients were taken at the initial visit, and before and immediately after each laser or IPL session by using a digital camera (we used Canon PowerShot A360) equipped with a special dermoscopic objective (Dermlite Photo, 3GEN LLC, San Juan Capistrano, CA, USA). Each picture was stored in a digital database with the aim to record each treatment performed.

Then, in our routine practice, dermoscopy has proved to be accurate in predicting and determining any damage and adverse events, and the dermoscopic examination resulted in a mandatory follow-up clinical session 4–6 weeks after treatment for all NMSCs treated with lasers and IPL-PDT.

Moreover, thanks to this precise iconographic documentation, the patients were able to observe and appreciate the achieved results, also because in an interval of 4–6 months of treatment they often did not remember exactly what the initial

---

The contents of this book are partially based on the Italian language edition: "*The Usefulness of Dermoscopy in Laser and IPL Treatments*", Domenico Piccolo, © DEKA M.E.L.A Srl 2012.

© Springer Nature Switzerland AG 2020

D. Piccolo et al., *Quick Guide to Dermoscopy in Laser and IPL Treatments*, https://doi.org/10.1007/978-3-319-41633-5_15

situation was and therefore they were really surprised seeing all the clinical and dermoscopic images of their treatment history. This obviously contributed to their satisfaction in both the economic and time investment they made to improve their condition.

In conclusion, at the end of this *Quick Guide to Dermoscopy in Laser and IPL Treatments*, we would like to underline that dermoscopic examination has proven to be a versatile, simple, and effective tool in dermatologic clinical practice, and we cannot but highly recommend its adoption as part of the routine protocol.

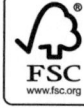

MIX
Papier aus verantwortungsvollen Quellen
Paper from responsible sources
FSC® C105338

If you have any concerns about our products,
you can contact us on
ProductSafety@springernature.com

In case Publisher is established outside the EU,
the EU authorized representative is:
Springer Nature Customer Service Center GmbH
Europaplatz 3, 69115 Heidelberg, Germany

Printed by Libri Plureos GmbH
in Hamburg, Germany